Technique in the Use of Surgical Tools

foreword by

Stephen L. Wangensteen, M.D.
Professor and Head
Department of Surgery
Health Sciences Center
The University of Arizona
Tucson, Arizona

TECHNIQUE IN THE USE OF SURGICAL TOOLS

Robert M. Anderson, M.D.

College of Medicine
Department of Surgery
Health Sciences Center
The University of Arizona
Tucson, Arizona

Richard F. Romfh, M.D.

Bellingham, Washington

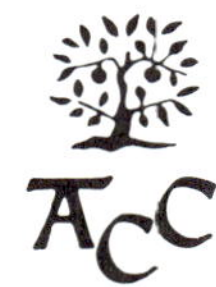

APPLETON-CENTURY-CROFTS/New York

Copyright © 1980 by APPLETON-CENTURY-CROFTS
A Publishing Division of Prentice-Hall, Inc.

All rights reserved. This book, or any parts thereof,
may not be used or reproduced in any manner without written
permission. For information, address Appleton-Century-Crofts,
292 Madison Avenue, New York, N.Y. 10017.

82 83 84 / 10 9 8 7 6

Prentice-Hall International, Inc., London
Prentice-Hall of Australia, Pty. Ltd., Sydney
Prentice-Hall of India Private Limited, New Delhi
Prentice-Hall of Japan, Inc., Tokyo
Prentice-Hall of Southeast Asia (Pte.) Ltd., Singapore
Whitehall Books Ltd., Wellington, New Zealand

Library of Congress Cataloging in Publication Data
Anderson, Robert M. 1920–
    Technique in the use of surgical tools.
    Includes index.
    1. Surgery, Operative. 2. Surgical
instruments and apparatus. I. Romfh, Richard F.,
1938–   joint author. II. Title.
[DNLM: 1. Surgical instruments. 2. Surgery,
Operative. W0500 A549t]
RD32.A58   617'.9178   80-17906
ISBN 0-8385-8842-5

Chapter 11, Perspectives on Sutures
    Copyright DAVIS + GECK, 1980

Photo Credit: William M. Anderson

PRINTED IN THE UNITED STATES OF AMERICA

CONTENTS

FOREWORD

There are numerous textbooks and monographs available to the student of surgery, but, to my knowledge, there never has been a useful treatise on technique in the use of surgical instruments or tools. Doctors Anderson and Romfh are very analytical in their approach to the use of each of the basic surgical instruments. Alternative methods and advantages and disadvantages of several techniques are described. The pros and cons of a variety of motions and manipulations are pointed out. Simple photographs very clearly illustrate the points the authors discuss. There are a variety of comments about operating room behavior and decorum which are proper and accurate. The poignancy of the aphorisms alone is enough to make the book worthwhile reading. In the past, surgeons have acquired their surgical skills in the use of surgical tools almost exclusively from individual staff surgeons or resident surgeons. This, of course, remains very important and will continue to be the major means of acquiring technical skills in the future. However, the surgical trainee studying the practical content of this book can gain considerably more insight into the use of the tools of his trade at a much earlier stage in his career. He can also apply alternative methods on occasion as the situation warrants. I believe that every surgical trainee should have the opportunity of reading this book with all of its wonderful tips.

Stephen L. Wangensteen, M.D.
Professor and Head
Department of Surgery
Health Sciences Center
University of Arizona
Tucson, Arizona

INTRODUCTION

Skilled surgical performance is facilitated by practicing the operative techniques shown to be optimal through mechanical analysis and clinical application. This monograph analyzes the mechanics of technical maneuvers with basic surgical tools; the analysis gives the student an appreciation of the advantages and disadvantages of the various options. We would encourage you, in developing your surgical technique, to select options dictated by rational mechanics rather than by loyalty to the judgment of superiors. Indiscriminately copying methods of prestigious institutions or teachers will include mimicking the weak points of experts.

Make sure your technique comes from analysis of mechanics rather than from prejudice or ego.

Your criteria for determining the best method should be *accuracy* and *security*, rather than speed and ease of performance. Speed and ease are by-products of accuracy and security, but the converse is not necessarily true. Many a poor operation has been performed in haste, motivated by the surgeon's urge to be speedy. Shortcuts that impair accuracy and security generally increase complications. The best surgeons appear to be deliberate. Their purposefulness and accuracy frequently allow them to complete procedures in less time than that taken by hurrying, unthinking technicians.

Practice produces skill. A well-planned operation composed of definite steps—each thoroughly practiced until securely performed—will result in a well-executed surgical procedure. Practice of each step is as important to the effectiveness of the surgeon as it is to a pianist or any other performing artist. Dedication to hours of thoughtful practice pays dividends to patients and artisan.

However, "Practice makes perfect" deteriorates to "Practice makes imperfect" when practice becomes the repetition of mistakes or cumbersome and inaccurate maneuvers. Mistakes become comfortable after they have been thoroughly practiced. Correction of a mistake in technique initially feels awkward and uncomfortable. Correction of poor technique always takes more practice than learning a good method in the first place.

Practice makes imperfect if it is repetition of mistakes.

Skilled surgical technique doesn't involve just skills of manual control. To be effective a surgeon must also control his personality and exercise leadership skills in his relationships with operating-room personnel. His techniques of self-control and self-discipline are extremely important, since his personality defects can leave a distinct imprint on his surgical results. In critical or hazardous operations, success is frequently inversely proportional to the irascibility of the surgeon. His ability to lead the surgical team and control the operation starts with his ability to control himself. Personality traits can be studied, practiced, and modified just as one can master the opening of a clamp or the holding of a knife.

Understand the mechanics involved in the use of your instruments. Use them in a manner that achieves accuracy and security. Strive for self-control and leadership with the same enthusiasm that you use to master your manual skills. Continue practice of these skills throughout your life, and your abilities as a surgeon will always move toward perfection.

We hope that you will use this book to improve your operative skills, not only to benefit the lives of your patients, but also to increase your fulfillment and that of your colleagues as you practice the healing art of surgery.

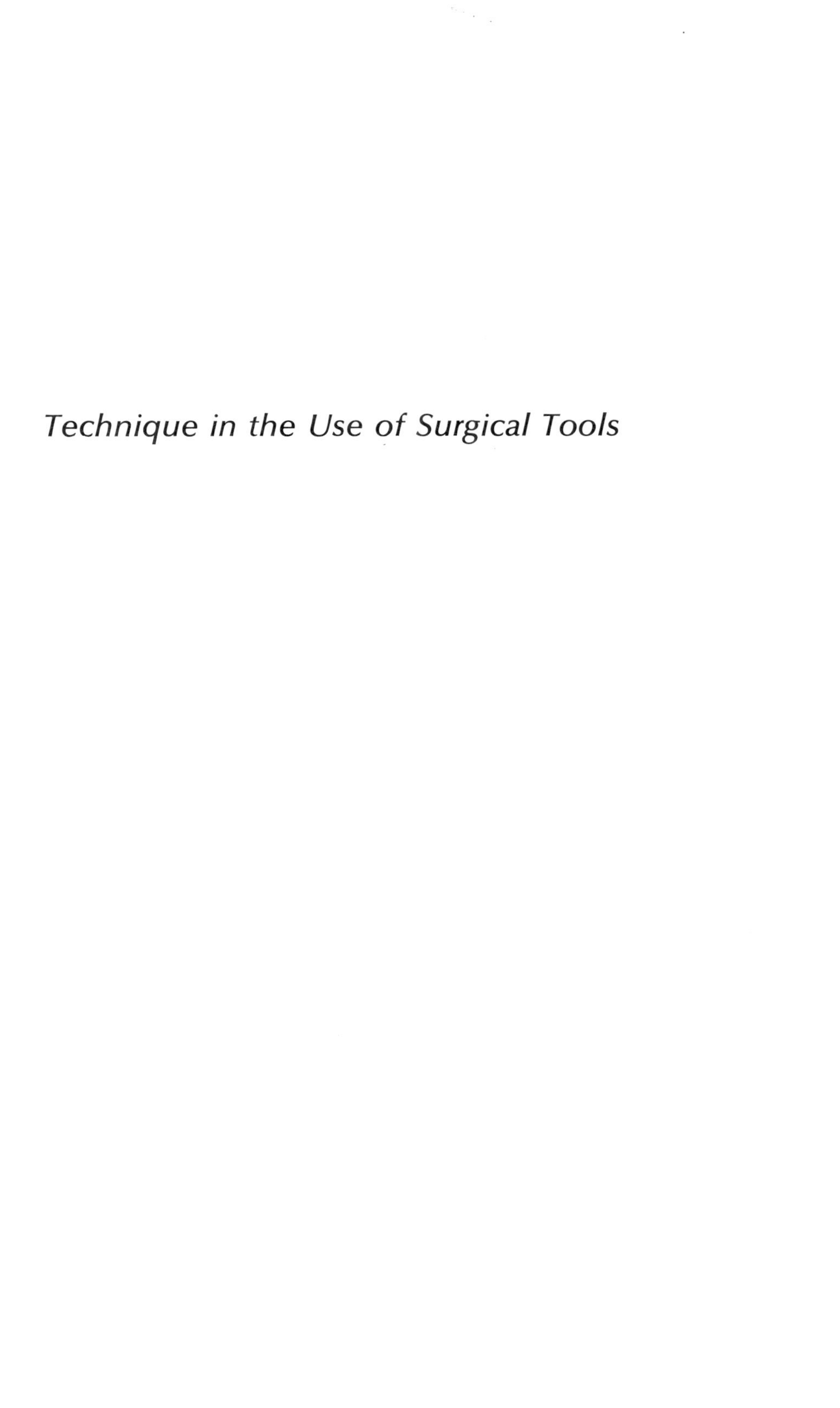

Technique in the Use of Surgical Tools

Chapter 1

The Scalpel

HOW TO HOLD THE SCALPEL

The scalpel can be held in three ways: the pencil grip, the finger-tip grip, and the palmed grip. Each of these grips can be used in making any incision, but each grip has its advantages and limitations. There are situations where one method of grasping can provide more accuracy and security than the other methods.

THE PENCIL GRIP. Grasping the scalpel like a pencil (Fig. 1) allows short, fine, precise incisions using the intrinsic muscles of the hand and the muscles of the forearm. The other ways of grasping the scalpel employ more gross wrist, arm, and shoulder motions and are less applicable to fine work. With the pencil position, the hand can be steadied by resting it on the patient to increase the precision of fine cutting.

The pencil grip is adaptable to backhand cutting (Fig. 2), allowing a change in cutting direction of 180° by reversing the direction of the blade without any change in arm position.

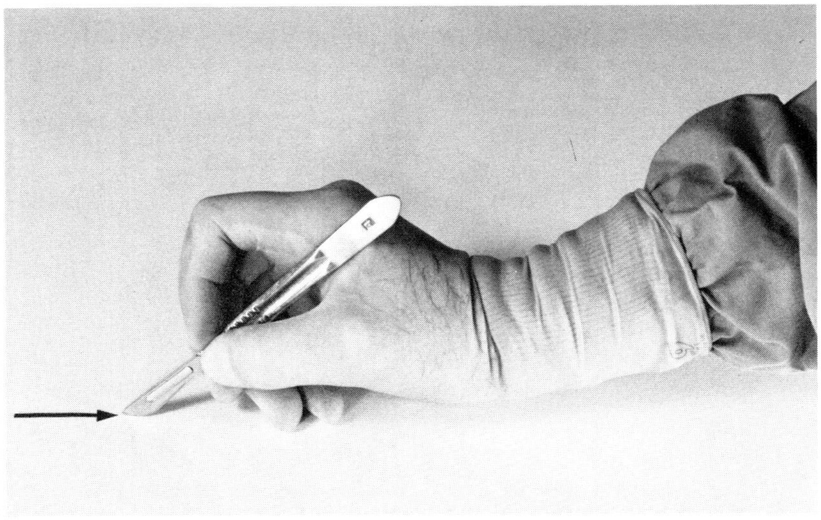

Figure 1. The pencil grip of the scalpel is useful for short, fine incisions.

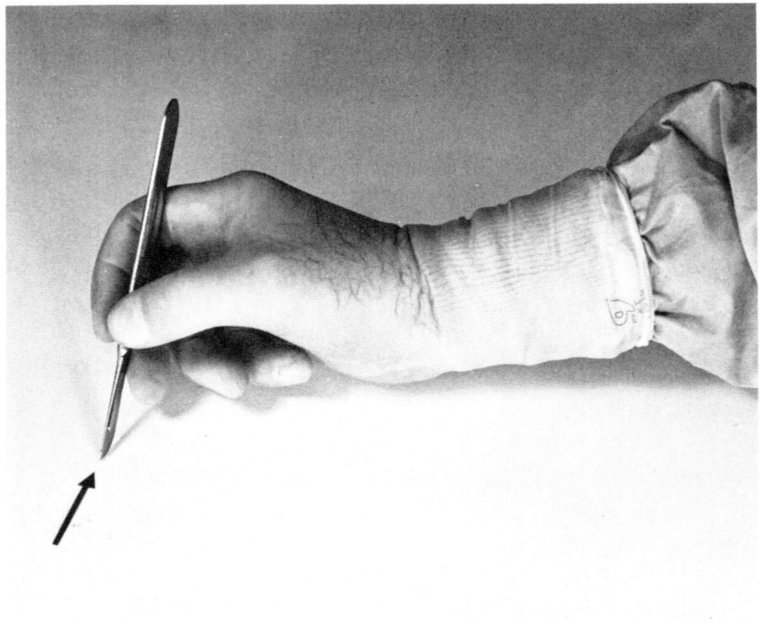

Figure 2. The pencil grip used in backhand cutting.

A good backhand is useful in both tennis and surgery.

For a given cut, the pencil position has 30–40° less ulnar deviation than the other two grips. Therefore, if an incision direction cramps the wrist in ulnar deviation with a fingertip hold, such as when cutting toward oneself, there is advantage in switching to a pencil position.

The major disadvantage of the pencil grip is that the scalpel is at a 30–40° greater angle to the tissue than with the other grips. This greater angle diminishes cutting edge contact, decreasing depth and direction control when making long arm motion incisions.

THE FINGERTIP GRIP. As shown in Figure 3, this grip has the advantage of placing maximum length of blade edge in contact with tissue. In making long incisions with arm motion rather than finger motion, the greater length of blade in contact with tissue, the less the depth variation with any change in cutting pressure. Any change in

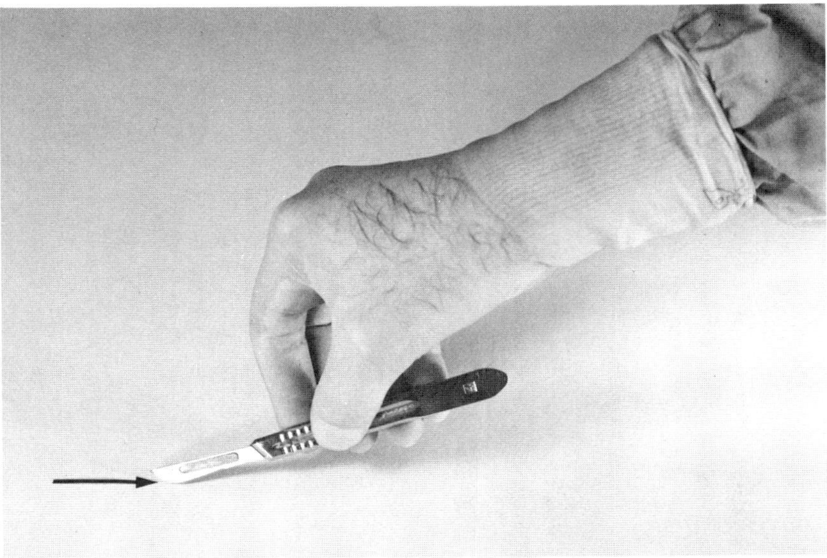

Figure 3. The fingertip grip allows maximum cutting edge contact for greater control in long incisions.

pressure distributed over a greater length delivers less pressure to each increment of tissue, with greater security in depth control. While making long incisions, direction control is enhanced by increasing the length of blade in the wound. The greater the length of tissue in contact with the scalpel, the more the walls of the incision resist minute or sudden changes in direction.

The finger grip has 30° less radial deviation of the wrist than the pencil position for the same incision. There is, therefore, advantage in switching to a fingertip grip whenever there would be cramping from radial deviation of a pencil position. An example is the making of a horizontal incision.

The fingertip grip has less dorsiflexion and radial deviation than the pencil grip.

THE PALM GRIP.   This grip (Fig. 4) has the advantage of being the strongest way to grasp a scalpel. This grasp is useful where great

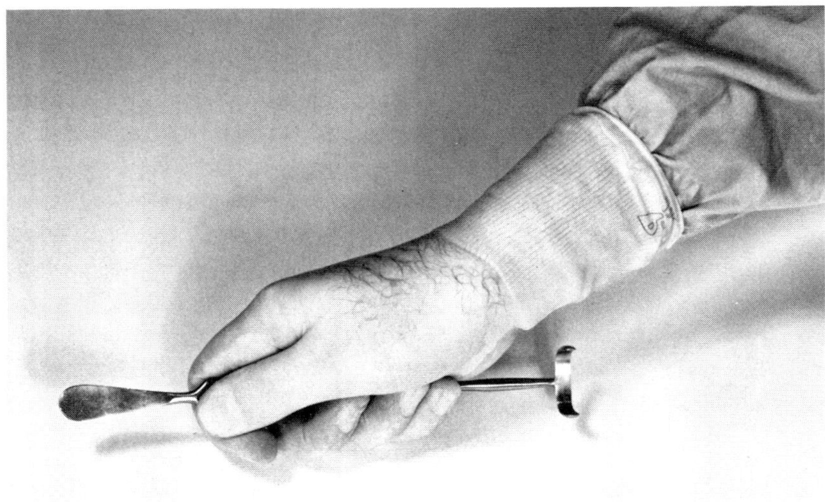

Figure 4.   The palm grip is useful when great pressure is needed.

pressure is needed and one requires a secure hold on specialized cutting tools such as a periosteal elevator, chisel, or osteotome.

Take advantage of all scalpel grips. Select the appropriate one by weighing the advantages and limitations of each hold for a given situation. Don't impede progress in the development of your technical skill by an arbitrary commitment to a single scalpel grip.

Take care not to mimic the mistakes of experts and
those you admire.

METHODS OF INCISING WITH A SCALPEL

There are four motions of the scalpel's cutting edge used in surgery: pressing, sliding, sawing, and scraping.

PRESS CUTTING. Press cutting (Fig. 5) is when the direction of pressure is the same as the direction of the motion of the blade as it incises the tissue. A stab is an example of a press cut, since the direction of blade motion and pressure are the same. To incise with a press cut, increase pressure on a stationary (nonsliding) blade until the bursting strength threshold of the tissue is exceeded; the knife then suddenly pops through. Depth control is not precise with pressing, because starting pressure is greater than the pressure needed to continue the path of the scalpel once the tissue begins to part. "Starting friction is greater than moving friction." With pressing, the difficulty in depth control is further accentuated when the outer layer of tissue has a greater bursting threshold than the deeper layers.

Use stab wounds in surgery, but refer to them as "incisions" in your operative reports.

In making stab wounds, depth control can be improved by exposing a limited amount of knife blade, by using a finger as a "bumper," and by resting the knife hand against the patient.

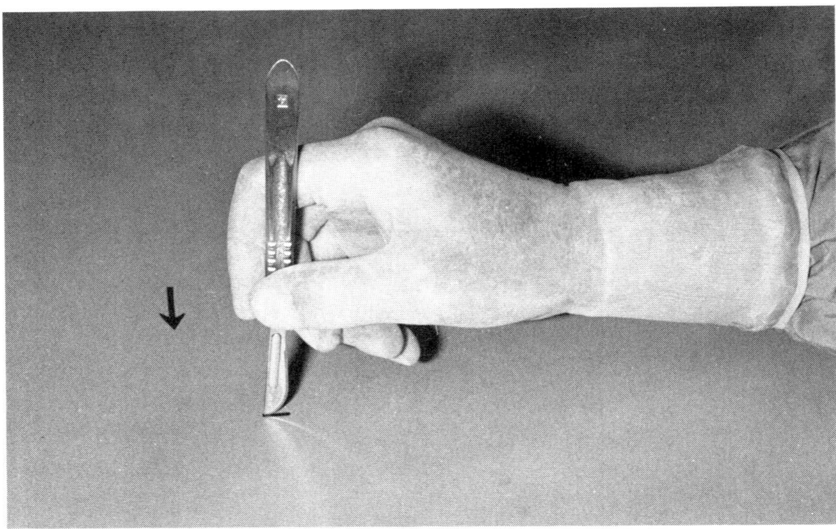

Figure 5. In press cutting, there is identical direction of pressure and of blade motion.

With press cutting, wounds are well controlled in length and direction. The length of a stab wound is exactly the width of the scalpel blade, and the direction is in line with the plane of the blade. Thus, press incising is useful where depth control is not critical. A stab can be used to open fluid-filled structures where, once the wall has been penetrated, the fluid provides space for the blade to decelerate and stop.

Appropriate uses of press cutting include the making of cannulation incisions in atria and the aorta during heart operations, and the incision and drainage of abscesses. Press cutting is useful when cutting sutures in the secondary opening of a recently closed wound. The pressure to pop the sutures is less than that required to cut the surrounding tissue. Thus, transection of the sutures by pressing with the knife blade occurs without the hazard of making a new parallel incision.

Press cutting is not applicable to situations such as making a transverse incision half the circumference of a small vessel. As soon as such a cut is started, the blade will go completely through the structure. The usefulness of press cutting is limited by the "all or none" quality of depth.

SLIDE CUTTING. A slide cut is made by sliding the knife blade on its cutting edge while exerting a sub-bursting pressure on the tissue (Fig. 6). In contrast to a press cut, where the direction of pressure and motion of the scalpel are the same, the motion (d, Fig. 6) is at a right angle to the direction of scalpel pressure (p, Fig. 6). Depth control with a slide cut is precise, since bursting pressure is never exceeded. The depth is determined by the amount of sub-bursting pressure exerted, length of blade distributing that pressure, and the resistance to cutting of the tissue being incised. The lighter the pressure and the more knife edge in contact with the tissue, the shallower the cut. Accuracy of depth control, associated with precise direction and length control, makes the sliding cut the most applicable of the scalpel motions.

Slide cutting allows great depth control.

SAWING. Sawing is merely "to-fro," or push-pull, slide cutting. Sawing has the unique feature of allowing a cut to be continued deeper

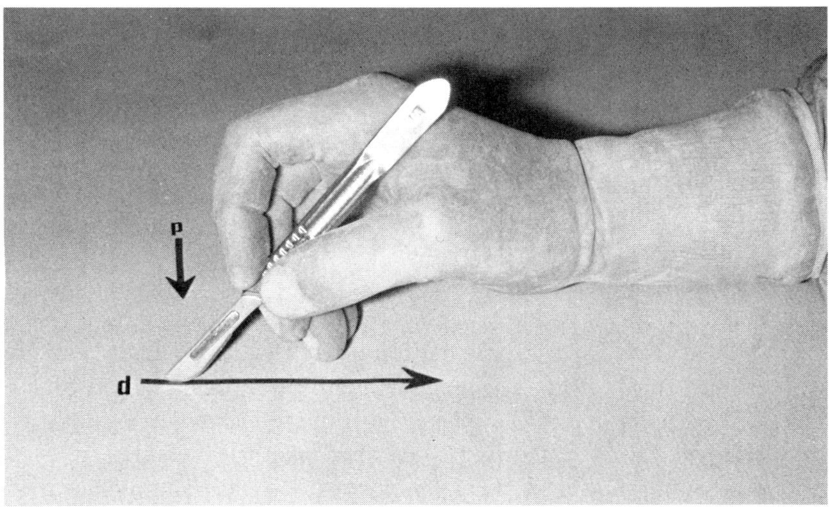

Figure 6. In slide cutting, blade motion (d) is at a right angle to scalpel pressure (p).

than a single slide cut, without the need for removing and reinserting the blade into the wound. The sawing motion is useful when cutting a freehand split thickness skin graft or for tailoring a posterior flap with a long knife during a below-the-knee amputation.

Sawing is usually for carpenters cutting wood, but occasionally for surgeons cutting patients.

One defect limits the usefulness of sawing with a scalpel in surgery. If a slip occurs while sawing down in a wound, the push portion of the "to-fro" motion will plunge the knife into the patient, whereas a simple slide cut would slip the knife out into the room. Sawing is hazardous where structures deep to the tissue being cut are in jeopardy if a slip occurs while pushing.

If you slip, slip into the room, not into the patient.

SCRAPING. Scraping (Fig. 7) is the cutting motion done by exerting a sub-bursting pressure while moving the scalpel perpendicular to both the edge of the blade and the direction of the pressure. Scraping is the method used in shaving whiskers. Since scraping will not cut the layer beneath the knife edge, it is a precise way to separate layers of tissue without the hazard of "buttonholing" that easily occurs from push cutting or slide cutting.

The accuracy of tissue layer separation gives scraping many surgical applications. The scraping motion promotes facility in developing pouches for prosthetic devices such as cardiac pacemakers and breast implants. Scraping eases the preparation of skin flaps during mastectomy and separation of fascial planes in reconstructive surgery.

A scraping motion of the scalpel gives security from perforation of serous surfaces while separating pleural, pericardial, and peritoneal adhesions. The same motion is used to elevate periosteum.

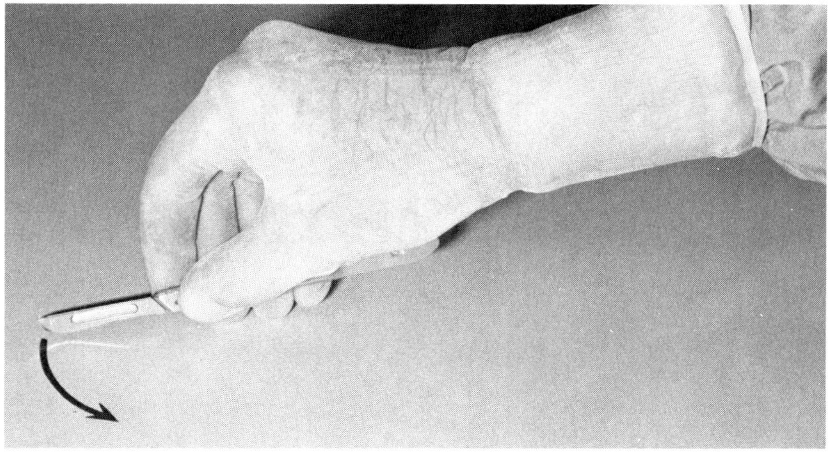

Figure 7. Scraping motion is perpendicular to both blade edge and pressure.

USE OF THE SCALPEL TO MAKE INCISIONS

Making a skin incision illustrates so many technical essentials in the use of a knife in general, and slide cutting in particular, that it warrants a detailed description. To have an incision turn out the way it was envisioned requires methods that give control over determining the location, length, direction, contour, depth, and cross-section configuration of the wound.

PLAN BEFORE CUTTING. Establish starting and stopping landmarks with the patient in a neutral position, to compensate for any skin distortion caused by a nonneutral position. For example: To make a straight median-sternotomy incision from the suprasternal notch to the xiphoid, the patient's head needs to be facing directly forward. If the incision is made with the head to one side, a straight cut will have a "hockey-stick" bend at the cephalad aspect of the wound after the head returns to a neutral position. After the incision is made in a neutral position, the head may be turned to give better exposure to deeper layers without compromising the ultimate cosmetic result.

In middle-aged women always cut parallel to a natural crease, never parallel to a wrinkle.

Landmarks are established using natural skin marks, such as freckles, blemishes, or wrinkles; or by making artificial marks at the proposed beginning and end of an incision. One method of artificial marking is to press the tip of a closed hemostat against the skin with enough force to cause a slight indentation. Such indented marks will be no more permanent than the marks left on the thighs from sitting on a cane chair. If desired, the entire contour of an incision can be pressure marked by exerting pressure on a piece of suture material stretched over the proposed incision site.

When cosmetic appearance is critical, starting and stopping marks as well as contour planning may be made with a skin-marking pen, using nontatooing dyes. A marking pen can also be of benefit in placing crosshatch marks across a proposed incision to allow accurate alignment of the skin at the time of closure. The use of scratch marks from the back of a scalpel to outline or crosshatch a proposed incision has the disadvantage of occasionally leaving permanent unsightly marks or keloids. Permanent marks, as well as being ugly, permanently advertise any inaccuracy of skin alignment by the surgeon.

STABILIZE THE SKIN DURING EXECUTION OF AN INCISION. To cut in the desired direction while preventing a jagged wound from redundant skin in the path of the blade, smooth out the surface by stretching the skin tightly. Both lateral and longitudinal tension are necessary to create a smooth surface.

In most cases the surgeon should be the only one touching and stretching the skin during the incision. If the surgeon uses an assistant to help place tension on the skin, neither person has any accurate measurement of the tension being exerted by the other. If the assistant is exerting more tension on one side than the surgeon on the other, a straight cut with the scalpel will result in a curved incision bowed toward the surgeon when the two relax. The surgeon can accurately know that his incision is going straight when he exerts tension with his thumb on one side and his other fingers opposite. His proprioceptive senses will allow him to equalize the tension on the two sides, thus preparing an undistorted surface for accurate incising.

Don't use your assistant to distort the skin.

Figure 8 shows the position of the assisting left hand. Tension is exerted in direction c-e, and c-e', resulting in longitudinal vector forces d-e and d'-e', and lateral vector forces c-d and c-d', so that the cutting surface can be stretched and the incision separated with the force c-e and c-e'.

During the incision, as the knife blade moves farther and farther from the assisting hand, the vector forces c-d and c-d' become smaller, while d-e and d'-e' become greater. At a certain distance, forces c-d and c-d', which have been separating the skin edges to allow visualization of the depth of the incision, are so small that the knife blade edge is no longer seen. At this point, cutting should stop and the assisting hand should be repositioned closer to the scalpel, so that vectors c-d and c-d' again become great enough to expose the depth of the parting tissue.

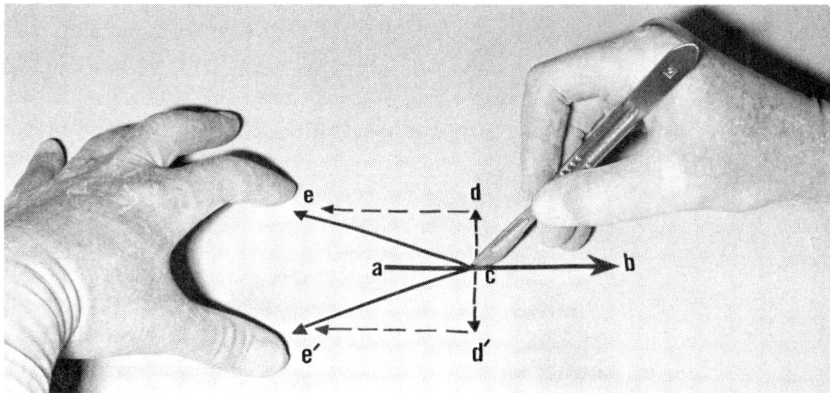

Figure 8. The surgeon's assisting left hand, with thumb and other fingers on opposite sides, provides a stretched, undistorted surface for incision. See text explication of vectors.

If you can't see the cutting edge of the scalpel you are operating by Braille.

Do not advance the assisting hand beyond the knife edge, as the vector forces d-e and d'-e' will be reversed in such a way as to wrinkle the skin beneath the knife and eliminate the benefit of longitudinal tension. When stopping to advance the assisting hand, do not remove the knife blade from the wound; there will then be no problem of trying to reinsert it at the exact stopping point. Removing and reinserting the scalpel can cause a small jog in the incision each time the assisting hand is advanced.

In making a curved incision, take care not to make any abrupt change in direction at the stopping points. In making long incisions, such as a thoracotomy wound, the assisting hand will need to advance three or four times to keep tension on the skin and to allow observation of the cutting edge of the knife blade throughout the course of the incision.

DEPTH CONTROL OF THE SKIN INCISION. It is ideal to cut completely through the skin with the first pass of the knife blade, thus assuring the best possible perpendicular skin edges for closure of the wound (Fig. 9b).

Be bold in all sure things.

If the skin is partially transected (Fig. 9c) a V-shaped groove will be formed by the superficial layers separating. The bottom of the V will fill with blood, making it impossible to observe the exact apex of the V for continuation of the incision. Frequently, the next incision which completes the skin transection will be slightly away from, though parallel to, the apex of the V-groove created by the first incision (Fig. 9d). If you can't see the cutting edge of the scalpel you are operating by Braille.

To assure proper depth control, use a slide cut. Position the knife

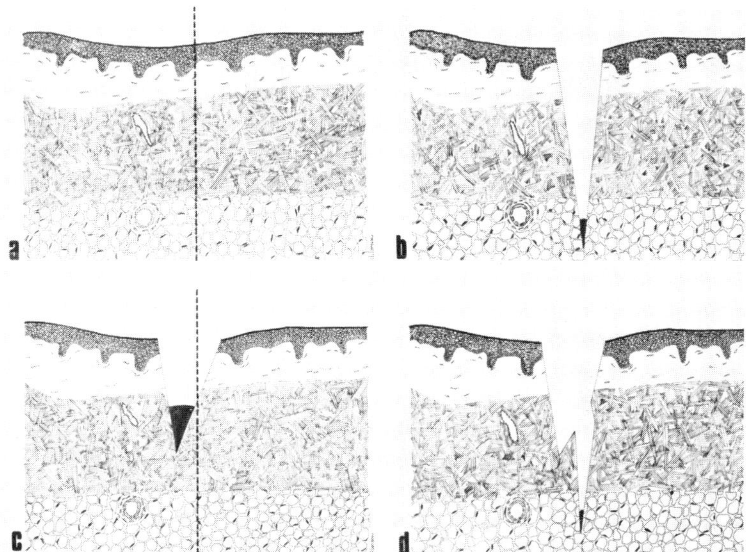

Figure 9.   Incisions. (A) Desired line of incision through skin. (B) Adequate first incision completely through skin, assuring clean perpendicular edges for wound closure. (C) Inadequate first incision, with skin only partially transected. (D) Jog in line of incision caused by noncontinuous second cut.

blade, exert sub-bursting pressure and draw the blade as described under "sliding incisions." As the skin begins to part, increase pressure until the edge of the blade is transecting a small amount of underlying fat. Adequate depth will usually be reached by the time the incision is 1.5–3 cm in length. Starting an incision with a press cut instead of a slide cut results in uncontrolled depth. Continue the incision while increasing or decreasing the pressure necessary to keep the blade at the proper level. One and one half to three centimeters of incision at each end will not be full thickness. Complete these two areas, holding the scalpel in the pencil position, to open precisely the corners of the wound and avoid the problem of jagged skin edges.

WHERE TO WATCH.   Focus your attention on the incision behind the scalpel blade to determine the amount of pressure adjustment needed to continue at the proper depth. To continue in a straight line, focus your attention upon the segment already cut, rather than on the destination. The same applies to a curved incision; focus on the segment already made in order to continue the desired curve.

While driving a car, watch where you are going; while making an incision, watch where you have been.

DIRECTION. When a minor deviation from the preconceived direction of the first part of the incision occurs, deviating the opposite way to correct it may compound the problem.

Take, for example, a minor deviation in direction at the beginning of the incision, as shown in Figure 10. The incision was planned to extend from Point 10a to Point 10b. After making half of the incision, the surgeon discovered that the direction of the first portion was off course. Correcting the direction to terminate at Point 10b would result in an esthetically poor "hockey-stick" incision, making it obvious to the patient and all observers that the incision was not created as planned.

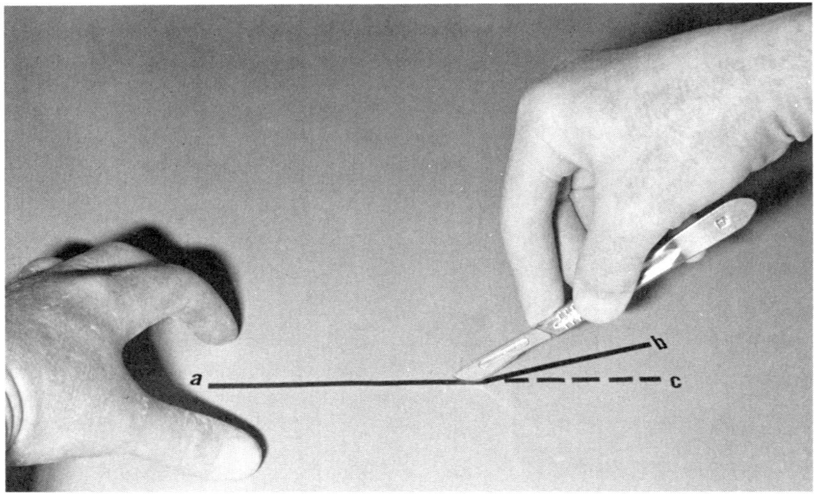

Figure 10. Though the incision A–B was planned, once the cut is off course, continue to (C) to avoid a "hockey-stick" correction.

However, when you discover that the incision is slightly off course, continue on in a straight line to Point 10c to achieve a satisfactory cosmetic scar. If Point "a" is in the midline and Point "c" is far from the midline, the patient will not wonder whether his surgeon was hung over from the night before as with a "hockey-stick" correction, but instead will think: "My, how straight my surgeon can cut. I wonder what anatomic circumstance in my operation required a slightly oblique incision."

ATTITUDE OF THE KNIFE BLADE DURING THE SKIN INCISION.

To prevent slicing the skin edges, keep the scalpel blade perpendicular to the skin surface. When the surface is curved, there is a tendency to keep the knife blade perpendicular to the floor instead of to the skin surface where the incision is being made.

Keep the scalpel face perpendicular to the patient, not perpendicular to the floor.

For instance, when making a standard right thoracotomy incision, starting from the back, the knife blade is horizontal or parallel to the floor, but perpendicular to the skin surface, and the surgeon's hand is in pronation. As the incision is extended up onto the patient's side, the knife blade goes from oblique to perpendicular with relation to the floor, and the hand moves from extreme pronation to moderate pronation, but the knife blade remains perpendicular to the skin surface throughout the incision. When the incision is extended across the side to the front of the chest, the knife blade goes from perpendicular to the floor to almost parallel again, and the surgeon's hand moves from pronation through the neutral position to slight supination. Again, throughout the entire incision, the knife blade remains perpendicular to the skin surface. This 180° change in attitude of the knife blade must occur gradually in order to make a perpendicular incision throughout the length of the wound.

INCISING THE SUPERFICIAL FASCIA.

This technique differs from cutting skin, since there is no cosmetic benefit to cutting in one uninterrupted motion. Shorter interrupted strokes allow pauses to secure hemostasis and exposure. The pencil position of the blade is useful for the shorter strokes.

After completing the incision through the skin into the superficial fat, there are two advantages in transecting the superficial fascia directly in line with skin incision. First, it assures viability of skin edges. The blood supply to the skin could be placed in jeopardy with any undermining between the skin and superficial fascia. Second, making the fascial incision directly in line with the skin promotes accurate closure, since accurate approximation of the fascia aligns the skin in such a way as to relieve tension on the skin sutures. In making an incision, act as though the superficial fascia belongs to the skin.

OTHER CUTTING TOOLS

Besides a variety of knife blade configurations, there are other cutting instruments, such as chisels, osteotomes, periosteal elevators, meniscus knives, bone and urterine curettes, strippers, dermatomes, and saws for special purposes. Just as with the scalpel, the best technique for using each of these instruments is the one that prevents slipping beyond the desired incision.

With bone-cutting chisels and osteotomes the most controlled cut is the one induced by a hammer or mallet. The least controlled cut with chisels and osteotomes is made by pushing. These cutting instruments are held in a secure palmed grip in the left hand to prevent them from changing direction from the desired course or from going deeper than determined by the magnitude of the mallet stroke (Fig. 11).

The depth of a slip from a push is almost unlimited, whereas a tap from a mallet causes a cutting instrument to go a precise predetermined depth.

The most delicate curette draw cut is made in soft tissue, such as endometrium, by finger and hand motion, with the instrument held like a scalpel in a pencil grip (Fig. 12). Better controlled than pushed

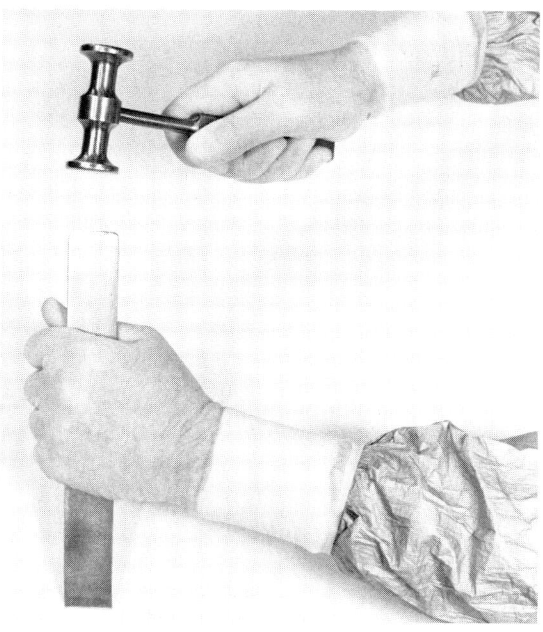

Figure 11. The bone cutting chisel, held in a palmed grip, is tapped by the mallet to achieve the desired direction and depth of cut.

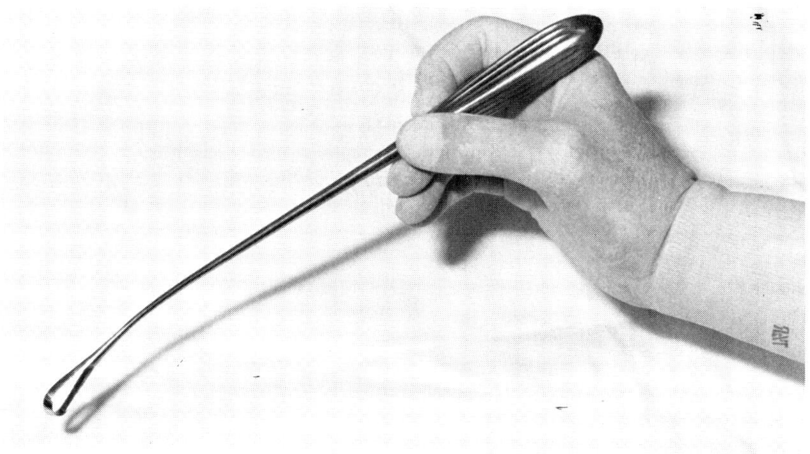

Figure 12. The curette, held in a pencil grip, makes a delicate draw cut in soft tissue.

strokes with a curette are back-and-forth rotating motions or pulling strokes, which eliminate the possibility of slipping deeper into the wound.

Bone power saws with rotational oscillation (e.g., Stryker) are designed so that the teeth move back and forth with such a short stroke that soft tissue tends to move with the teeth rather than be cut. Nevertheless, there is no absolute preference of the saw for bone. If you press the saw too firmly or leave the blade in contact too long against soft tissue, it will produce a cut. Such a hazard becomes manifest if you saw bones with the pressure on the blade in line with the cut when the undersurface is hidden from view. However, if you cut such an incision in increments by an up-and-down motion of the saw, you can remove that danger. Here, by pressing down on the blade perpendicular to the line of the cut, you can feel the blade penetrate the deep cortex and immediately release pressure. Then advance the blade in a shallower depth and again press to go through the next increment of the deep table.

The Stryker saw has limited blade radius, so to obtain maximal cutting depth do not encircle the gearbox with the right hand. Hold the motor in your left hand (Fig. 13) to provide direction attitude and stability. Then press on the gearbox with the heel of your right hand (Fig. 13) to obtain the desired pressure on the blade. You will be able to sense with your right hand the instant the blade pierces the deep cortex.

Bone saws which oscillate up and down (e.g., Sarns), instead of oscillating in a rotational direction, have a guide at the deep end of the blade that protects the underlying tissue (Fig. 14). It is necessary to separate the soft tissue beneath the bone before cutting, to provide a path for the guide and to prevent entrapment of the deep structures.

THE KNIFE IN SUMMARY

The knife can be held with three basic grips. The fingertip position offers the most accuracy and stability in making long incisions. The pencil position, using finger motion, is most accurate for short delicate maneuvers. The palm grip offers power for use with special cutting instruments, such as the periosteal elevator.

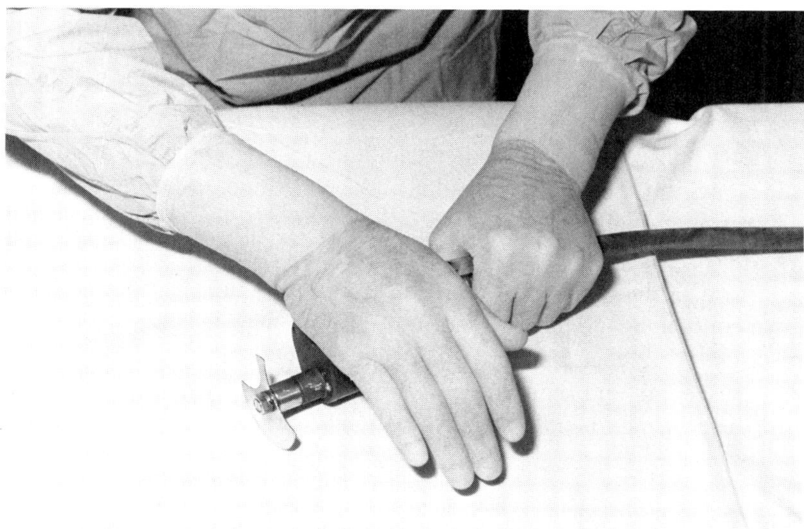

Figure 13. To utilize full blade radius of the Stryker bone saw, the right hand achieves desired blade pressure without encircling the gearbox. Holding the motor in the left hand provides stable direction.

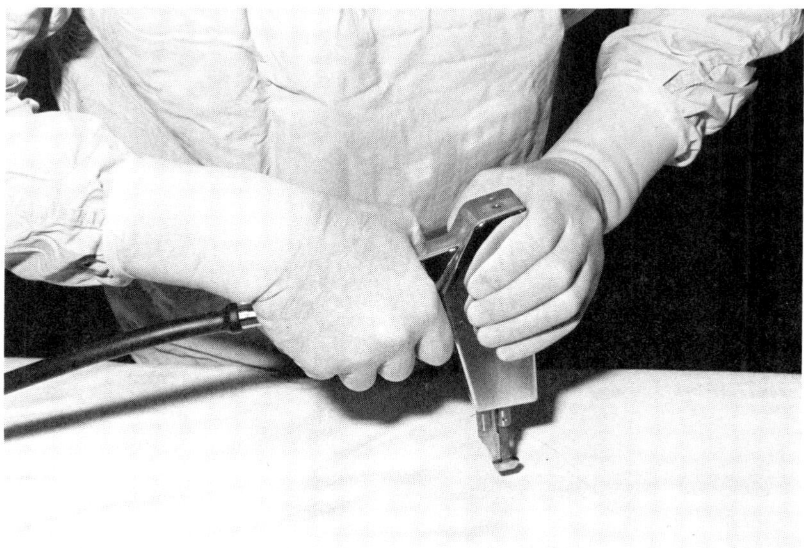

Figure 14. The Sarns bone saw, which oscillates up and down, has a guide at the deep end of the blade to protect underlying soft tissue.

There are four motions of cutting with a scalpel. Slide cuts give precise depth and direction control. Press cuts are useful in opening fluid-filled chambers; however, they are poorly controlled in depth. Scraping is the most accurate method of separating tissue planes. Sawing allows continuation of a cut without removing and reinserting the blade. Sawing is therefore useful in freehand skin graft removal; however, the push half of the motion is hazardous down in a wound.

Incising with a scalpel requires planning, with appropriate landmarks and skilled execution. Execution requires depth, direction, and length control, made possible not only by the proper selection of holding and cutting motions, but by using the assisting left hand effectively, watching and adjusting appropriately, and keeping the blade at the proper perpendicular attitude to the tissue.

There are so many things to think about, and it is possible to think of only one thing at a time. Complicated physical activity, to be done well, comes from automatic behavior, requiring no conscious thought. Such activity is made possible by repetitious concentration on one facet at a time.

Chapter 2

Scissors

Scissors should be so used to provide the most accuracy and control for the maneuver performed. Scissors can be used for sharp cutting and for blunt dissection.

Scissors are designed so that three force vectors are used in cutting: closing, shearing, and torque (Fig. 15). These forces are transferred from the hand to the shanks, then through a fulcrum to the cutting edges. The closing force is that which causes the blades to come together (Fig. 15a). Shearing is the force that pushes one blade flat against the other while closing (Fig. 15c). Torque is the force that rolls the leading edge of each blade inward to touch the other (Fig. 15b). Most scissors are designed so that the gripping motion of the right hand effectively combines these forces to result in precise cuts.

In cutting, direction control and accuracy depend upon the stability of the tissue between the scissor blades and the security of the operator's grip on the scissors. The wider the scissors are opened and the closer the tissue is to the fulcrum, the more the blades tend to push the tissue away, bunching it ahead of the shearing action of the blades. Thus, the more obtuse the angle between the blades when cutting, the less the scissors stabilize the tissue and the less accurate the cut.

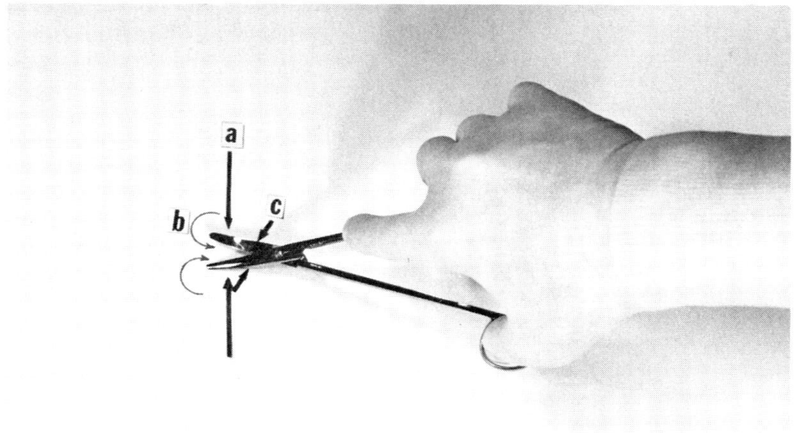

Figure 15. The gripping motion of the hand transfers three forces to the scissor blades: (A) Closing force; (B) Torque; (C) Shearing force.

Cutting nearer the scissor tips provides less closing force on the tissue but stabilizes the tissue more securely between the blades.

Scissors stabilize tissue between the blades and therefore cut flaccid tissue more accurately than can be done with a scalpel.

Gripping the Scissors

The grip that makes the best use of scissor design to apply the three force vectors will result in crisp, clean cuts. Scissors are most commonly held with the tips of the thumb and ring finger through the finger rings and with the index finger resting on the shanks near the fulcrum (Fig. 16). This grip provides the largest "tripod" and therefore gives the best stability for direction control. The normal grasping motion of this grip applies maximum shear, torque, and closing forces; and is, therefore, the grip that gives maximal control.

Don't operate like a cub bear, using paws instead of fingers.

Figure 17 shows the thumb and middle finger grip which allows the index finger to be used to support the sides of the shanks. The resulting three-point grasp creates a smaller tripod than the previous method and is, therefore, slightly less stable.

Figure 18 depicts the thumb-index finger grip, with the scissors held to cut in a forward direction. Such a grip uses only two-point direction control which may allow a cut to wander off course. Though closing force is strong, this grip applies the least shearing and torque forces of all the grips possible for forward cutting. With less shear and torque the blades will tend to "chew" rather than cut thick tissue cleanly.

Figure 19 shows the thumb-index finger grip used for cutting in a reverse direction. Such a grip applies three-point direction control with good lateral stability, but the shear and torque forces are virtually nonexistent. This reverse direction grip's main advantage lies in push cutting toward the operator.

The backhand grip (Fig. 20) is really a slight variation in the thumb-ring finger grip and is useful in cutting toward the right.

All grips discussed to this point provide strong closing force. The thumb-ring finger grip provides the best direction control, shear and

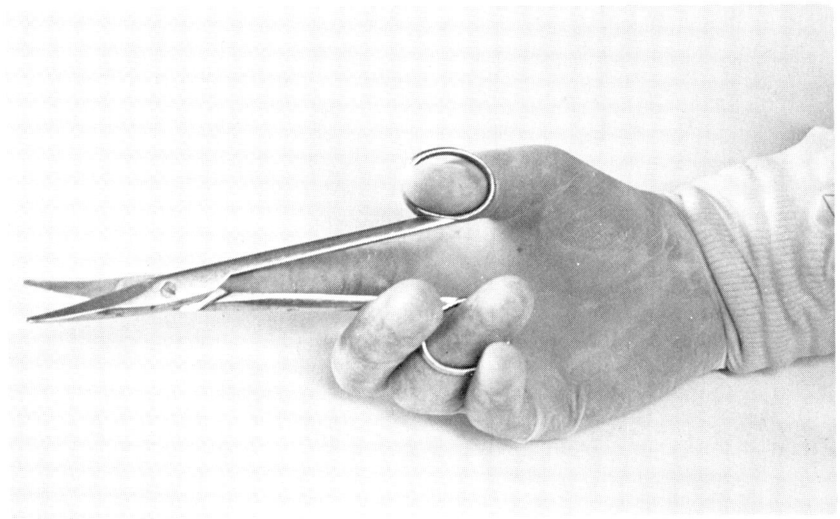

Figure 16. For maximal control, use a large "tripod" scissors grip: thumb and ring finger each through a finger ring, with index finger near the fulcrum.

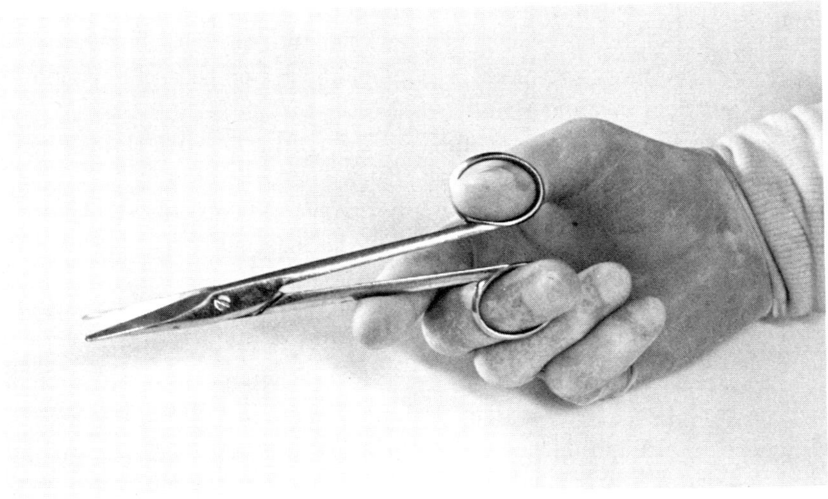

Figure 17. The smaller tripod of thumb and middle finger in finger rings and index finger beside the shank provides less stability than the grip shown in Figure 16.

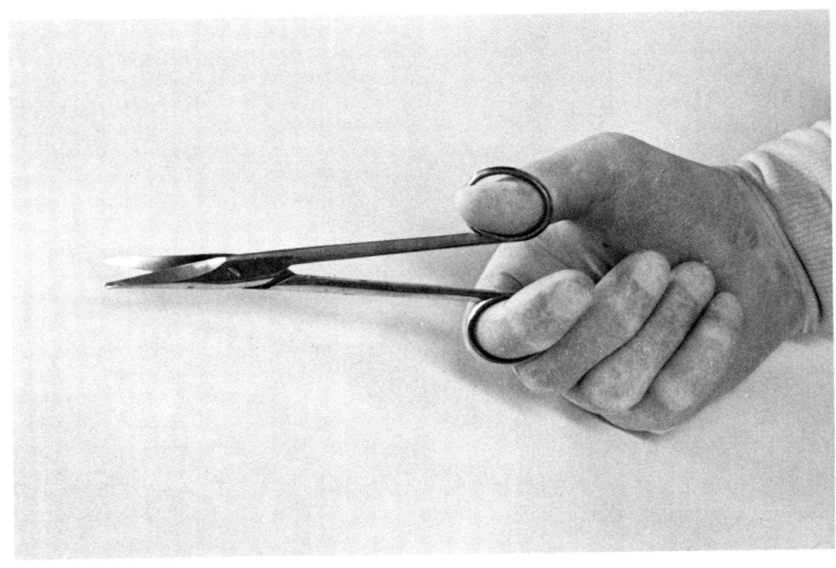

Figure 18. The thumb–index finger grip diminishes shear and torque.

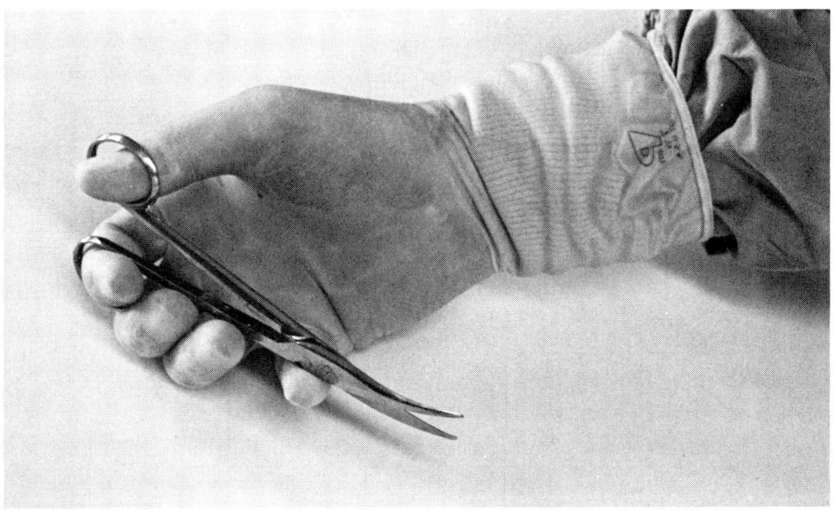

Figure 19. The thumb–index finger grip as shown gives good direction control in reverse push cutting.

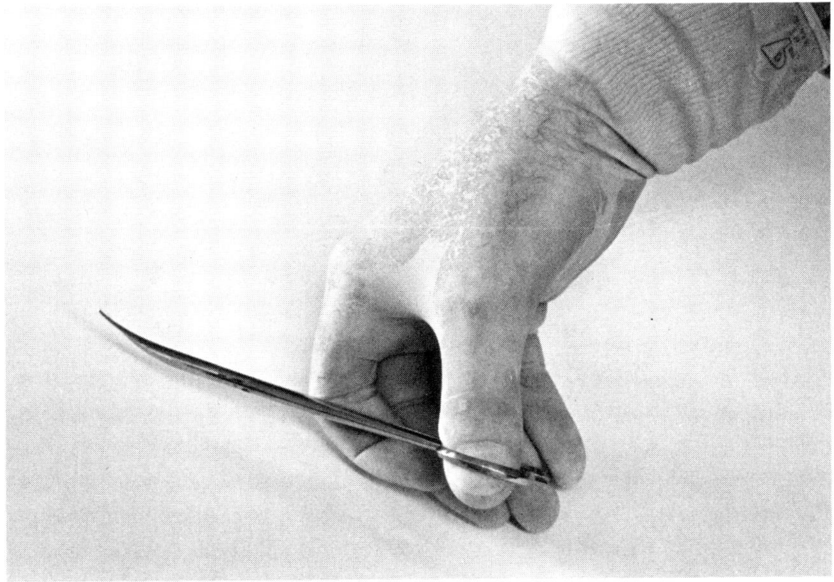

Figure 20. The backhand variation of the thumb and ring finger grip is for cutting to the right.

torque forces. For reverse cutting, the grip shown in Figure 19 is most stable in direction control. The other two grips, if used in reverse cutting, lose their directional stability.

The thenar eminence-ring finger grip shown in Figure 21 offers poor closing and opening forces. Although it does apply adequate shear force, torque is almost nonexistent. The weakened grasp and poor control in opening and closing the blades make this a clumsy method, without particular advantage; the grip is a surgical stunt. The difference between humans and other mammals is that humans have fingers instead of paws. The thenar method uses the hand as a paw. Another affectation of scissor grip (Fig. 22) is done without any fingers in the finger holes. Such a grip also is mere affectation, without application.

A surgical stunt or affectation is any maneuver that accomplishes nothing except to show how "cool" the operator is, man.

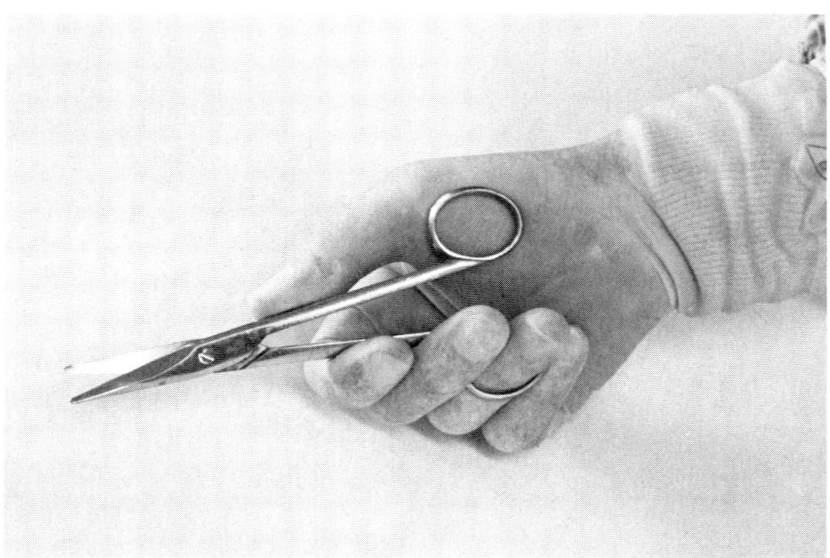

Figure 21. Using only one finger ring robs the scissors of closing and opening force and of torque, and trades control for showmanship.

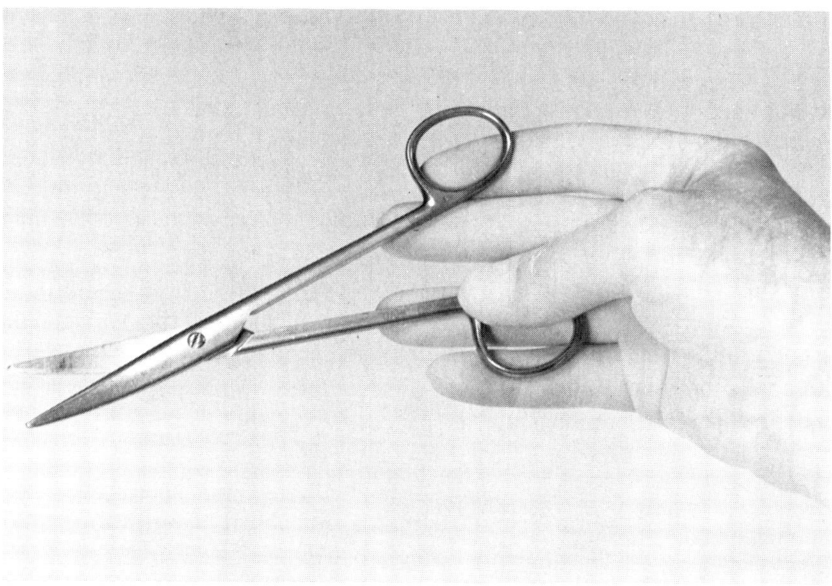

Figure 22. To spurn use of the finger holes (a practical design feature of scissors) is imprudent stage business in surgery.

Right-handed scissors are designed so that, with the palm down, the thumb blade is hinged beneath the finger blade. This blade arrangement allows the natural pushing of the thumb and pulling of the fingers in a gripping motion of the right hand to apply maximal shear and torque to the blades. When used in the left hand, the thumb blade is above, so that a grasping motion that pushes with the thumb causes loss of shear and torque forces. One can improve upon left-handed scissoring by using the awkward motion of pulling with the left thumb and pushing with the left ring finger in their respective finger rings (Fig. 23). Such motion will achieve improved shear and torque of the blades, but the push of the ring finger does not add useful torque to the blade's leading edge. If you are left-handed, consider either learning to cut with your right hand or procuring a pair of left-handed scissors.

Using right-hand scissors with the left hand is as awkward as wearing your pants backwards.

Hand, Arm, and Body Attitudes While Using Scissors

With the scissors grasped for maximal control, how should the hand be held while cutting? It can be held in pronation, in supination, or in any attitude between the two. While thinking of the hand position, consider what each position does to the arm, shoulder, and the rest of the body. Scissors held in a supinated hand while cutting horizontally, as in Figure 24, cause the elbow to be pressed firmly against the side. With the forearm in complete supination there is no ability to manipulate further in supination unless you lean to the right, push your trunk to the left with your elbow, and raise your left foot off the floor. To be mobile, use supination only where it can be used without needing further supination.

Don't let your elbow push you out of the operation.

Scissors held in the pronated hand (with the palm down), as in Figure 25, leave the elbow away from the body. The hand in pronation is still mobile in that it can be supinated 180° and by abducting the arm can be pronated 90° without any change in body position. The palm-down position, therefore, allows the greatest maneuverability of the scissors for horizontal cutting.

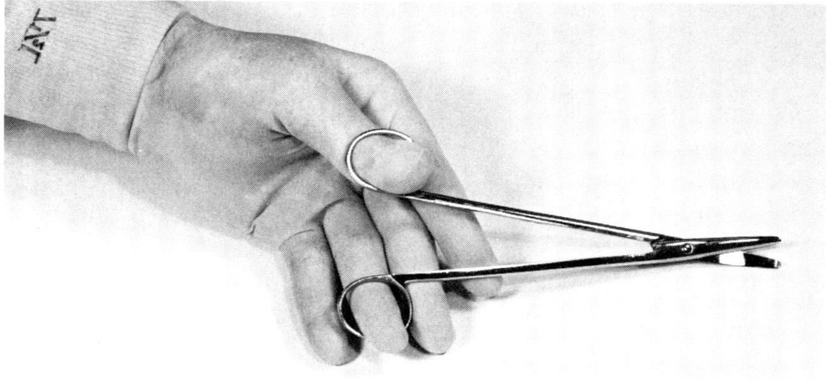

Figure 23. The left-handed use of scissors designed for the right hand reverses the pushing and pulling action of the shanks.

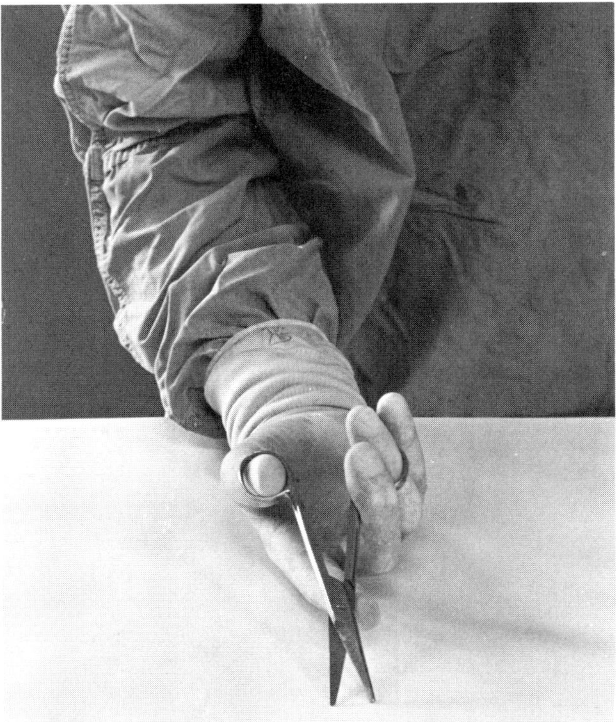

Figure 24. With hand and forearm supinated, adjustment can be made only in pronation.

Don't be boxed into a position of nonmaneuverability.

For vertical cutting the forearm is positioned midway between pronation and supination. The midway position allows maneuverability of 180° of pronation and 90° of supination.

Uses of Scissors

Scissors are used for both cutting and blunt dissection. In cutting, the scalpel yields two advantages to scissors. They can precisely cut flaccid tissue which cannot be held under tension, and they allow

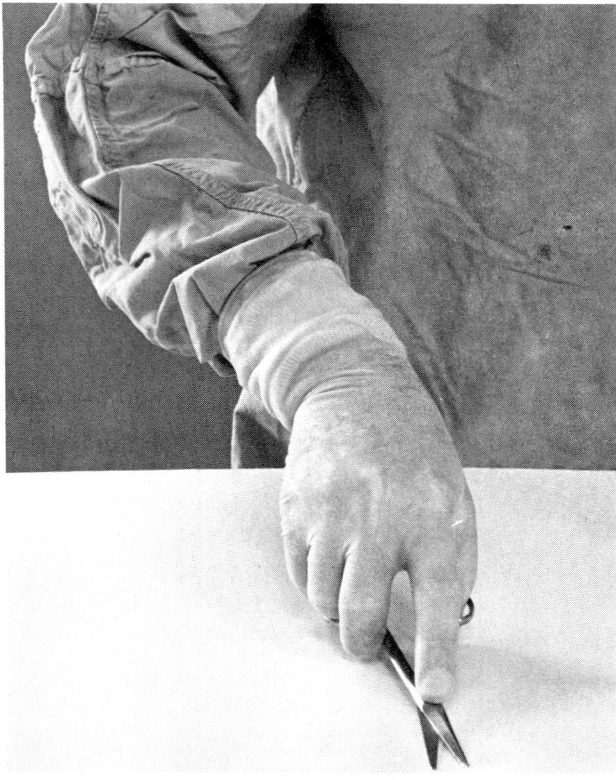

Figure 25. Holding scissors with the palm down allows adjustment by both pronation and supination.

excellent depth control. The flaccid tissue is stabilized between the blades and therefore allows excellent direction control. The scalpel has the advantage of incising through an intact surface, whereas scissors need an opening to insert the lower blade.

Scissors can be used to make three types of cuts: scissor-cuts, push-cuts, and chewed-cuts. With scissor-cutting, all three of the force vectors are important; with push-cutting, only two are significant. For push-cutting, the scissors are held with slightly opened blades. No closing force is used, but maximum, though static, shear and torque forces are exerted while the instrument is pushed through a sheet of tissue.

Chewing is crush-cutting caused by the lack of shear and torque. This results when the cutting edges of the blades are separated at the time of scissor closing and occurs when widely opened scissors push tissue ahead of the closing blades instead of cutting cleanly. Chewing results in ragged cuts of crushed tissue and can be avoided by using sharp instruments with optimal scissor grip. Chewing can also be avoided by cutting tissue nearer the tips rather than close to the fulcrum. Use just enough blade length to complete the desired cut. Chewing can be avoided when cutting thick tissue by taking several bites initiated with the tips rather than one large bite starting near the fulcrum of the scissors.

Push-cutting can open sheets of tissue accurately, e.g., pleura, peritoneum, and pericardium. In fascia and muscle, the push-cut follows the direction of the grain, producing excellent direction control. As starting resistance is greater than continuing resistance, there is advantage in starting and ending a push-cut with a short scissor-cut. Starting with a short scissor-cut will allow a push-cut to be initiated with less pressure. Ending the push-cut with a scissor-cut will provide greater control of the length of the cut without the possibility of slipping and going farther than intended. Start the push-cut with a short scissor-cut, stop the closing action with the blades held at an acute angle that contains the tissue layer, and continue the cut by pushing the scissors forward through the tissue. Terminate the push-cut by continuing with a scissor-cut to the proper end without pushing as the terminal scissor-cut is made.

Push-cutting is useful to both tailors and surgeons.

Suture Cutting

When cutting sutures, open the scissors wide enough to get a blade on either side of the suture without "past pointing." Opening the blades fairly wide does not commit you to use anything other than the tips of the scissors for cutting. To prevent inadvertent damage to deeper structures, don't lose sight of the blade tips beyond the suture.

Hold the scissor blades perpendicular to the suture being cut to keep the knot in view between the blades (Fig. 26), to assure that you cut at the right distance from the knot. You do not improve your view of the knot by lifting the shanks and looking beneath the blades (Fig. 27). Approaching the suture several inches from the knot, then sliding down the suture is a redundant maneuver. The method of turning scissors as a spacer while cutting, to give a short uniform free end, seems a good procedure for those with weak eyes or those with poor eye-hand coordination.

Metzenbaum scissors are great suture scissors. You, too, can afford the best.

If there are to be three half hitches on each knot, valuable time can be saved when the cutter brings the scissors into the wound during the third tie. The suture can then be cut deliberately and accurately,

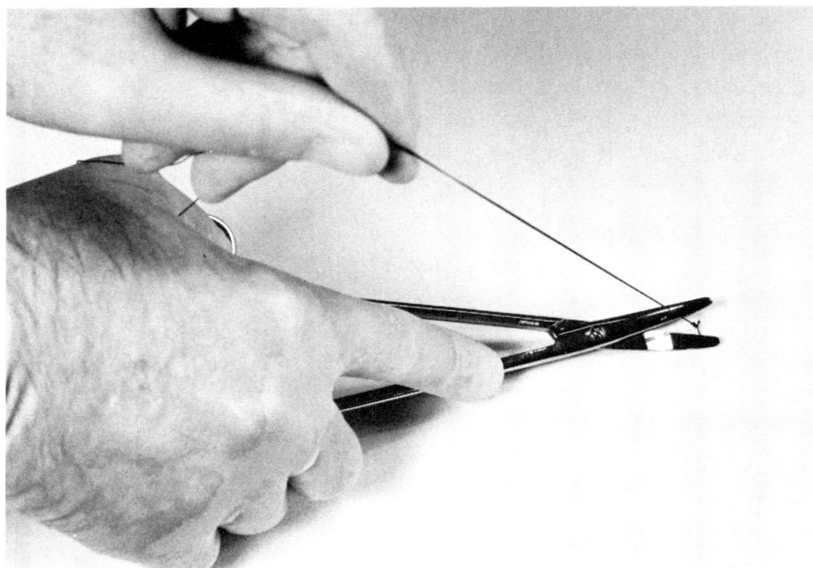

Figure 26. Cut a suture with the scissor blades perpendicular to the suture and with the knot in view between the blades.

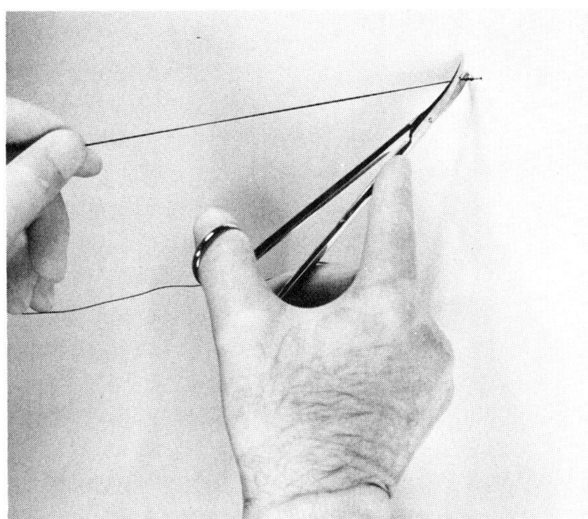

Figure 27. When cutting a suture, looking beneath the blades does not improve accuracy.

while saving time over the method where the scissors come in hurriedly after the knot is finished. Cutting with a hurried jabbing or snapping motion may tear the tissue if the scissors "misfire" and chew the ligature only partway through.

Save time by coming in early to cut the tie, then spend the time on deliberate and accurate cutting.

While cutting ligatures on a moving target it is best for the cutter to grasp the ligature in one hand and then cut with the other, thereby allowing coordination of the motions of his two hands. It is easier to coordinate the motions of one's own two hands, as one hand is sensing the movemen of the tissue and the other doing the cutting, than trying to synchronize with motion of a tie held by another person.

It is more difficult to synchronize cerebella than it is to synchronize tremors between your two hands.

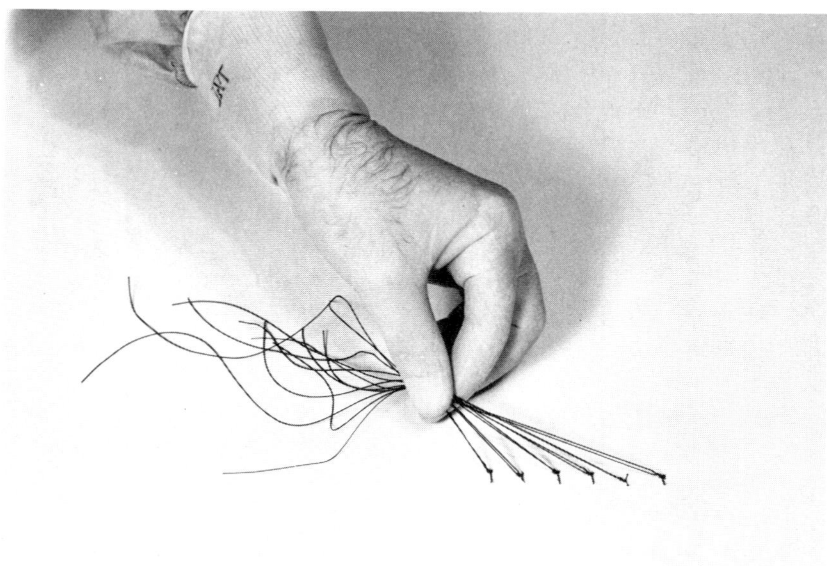

Figure 28. To cut a row of tied sutures, the left hand firmly holds taut sutures so that lengths are graduated, and so that the shortest and first to be cut is at the right.

When cutting a suture deep in a wound, or in critical situations, it is worthwhile to steady the scissor blades by using your left hand or a fixed part of the wound as a fulcrum.

If a row of sutures is tied prior to cutting, grasp the sutures with your left hand in such a way as to make each suture a different length, with the shortest one toward the right hand (Fig. 28). By firmly grasping the row of sutures in that position without letting them slip, you can apply perpendicular tension that will automatically tighten the suture being cut, while those already cut are held out of the way (Fig. 29). By holding sutures yourself, you can see best how to approach them with the scissors.

He who cuts, holds.

After cutting several sutures at a time, discard them by giving them to the instrument nurse, to avoid cluttering the field and confusing the procedure, When discarding a single cut suture, however, it will save time to toss it on the floor, where it will neither clutter the wound nor interrupt the activity of the instrument technician.

Discarding ligatures on the floor unclutters the wound, lessens the work of the scrub technician, and adds to the job security of the janitor.

Wire and pin cutting are done with special scissors and cutters. Before cutting, always grasp what will become the severed end of the wire or pin with a clamp, to avoid the hazard of producing a missile which could injure someone's eye (Fig. 30).

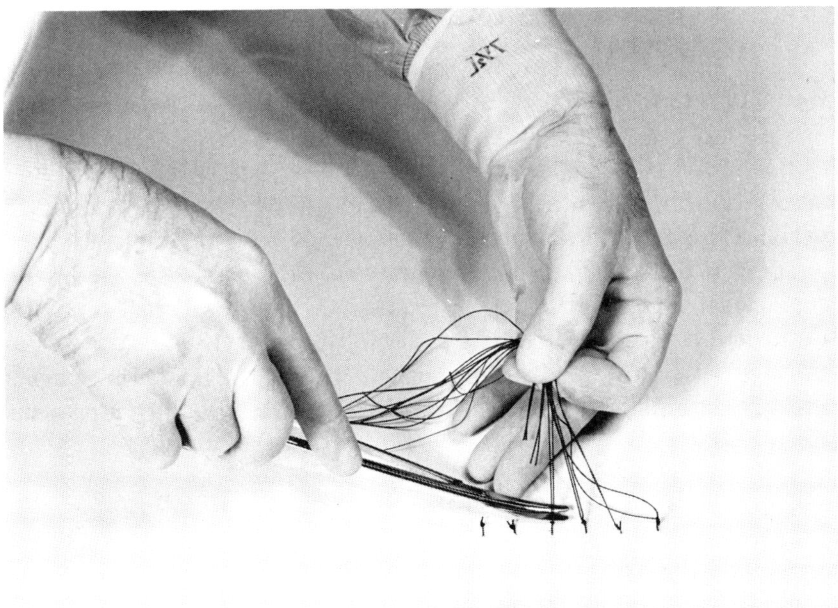

Figure 29. As tension is applied, the suture being cut is straightened while those already cut are no obstacle.

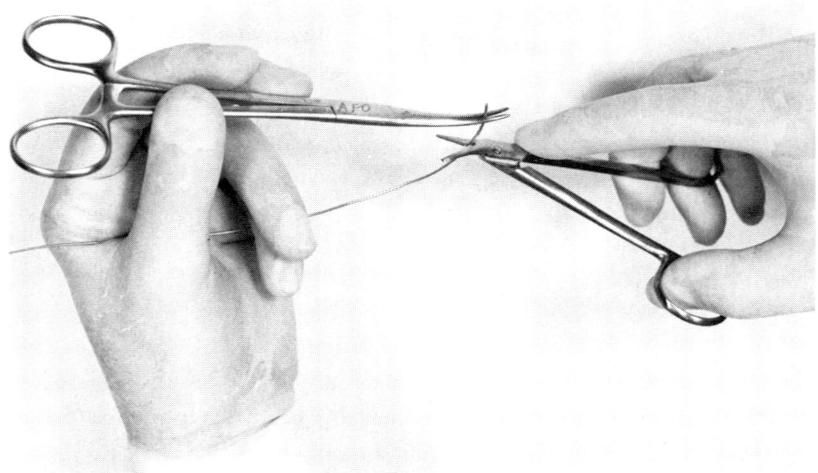

Figure 30.   Using a clamp to hold the end of a wire or pin before cutting avoids the risk of flying wire.

Blunt Dissection

As well as being excellent tools for sharp cutting, scissors with appropriate tips are ideal for blunt dissection by spreading, raking, or probing. Scissors have an added advantage over a clamp for blunt dissection, because alternating sharp and blunt dissection can be accomplished without changing instruments. Blunt dissection separates tissue layers held by cementing substance of less tensile strength than the layers themselves. The cementing substance can be either normal areolar tissue, as between fascial layers, or scar tissue from previous surgery.

In the blunt dissection of layers bound by scar tissue you will encounter hazard where the scar tissue traverses the cut in one of the layers. Blunt dissection of adhesions between layers proves risky when the adhesions have greater tensile strength than the bound layers. A scar may bind bowel to fascia or parietal pericardium to the heart with greater tensile strength than is present within the bowel or within the myocardium. Blunt dissection in these cases may be inappropriate and result in an unplanned enterostomy or entrance into the myocardium. It is therefore dangerous to blunt dissect where old scars traverse natural planes or where dense scar tissue is stronger than the structures it binds.

Most cutting and blunt dissection with scissors is under direct view. Blind scissor cutting and blunt dissection can sometimes be of great advantage and may be accurate and secure. Such blind dissection is done between well-established tissue planes in anatomic regions away from such critical structures as large vessels and nerves. Blind scissor dissection is an excellent method for opening a tunnel just beneath the dermis to insert a bovine heterograft when creating an arterial venous fistula.

Operating by Braille is often permissible with scissors, but never with the scalpel.

Blind scissor dissection can also be put to advantage while performing a breast biopsy through a small circumareolar incision. Often it is difficult to see the deep side of a breast lump; but, by palpation, using the left index finger as a guide, scissors can be used to circumscribe and remove the lump.

While exposing major blood vessels by blunt dissection with scissors, exercise care to avoid contusing the vascular wall or tearing small tributaries and branches. If scissors are used to spread parallel to a major vessel, concentrate on preventing any tearing of small side branches; whereas, if spreading is done perpendicular to the great vessel, direct your attention to preventing contusion of the wall or loosening of atheromatous plaques. Both methods, though having drawbacks, can be used if the inherent problems are understood.

Types of Scissors

Although you will find many sizes and shapes of scissors—each bearing the name of a famous surgeon—there are basically two types: those with straight blades and those with curved blades.

Scissors with curved blades offer directional mobility, visibility and the means to cut tissue in a smooth curve easily. The 15–20°

range of motion and visibility of structures over that found with straight scissors. Curved scissors are extremely useful deep in a wound where horizontal cutting with good visibility is desired. Straight scissors have a mechanical advantage for cutting tough tissue. In some situations, straight scissors can provide a more precise straight cut than the curved ones.

Curved scissors have 30–40° more mobility and visibility than straight ones.

Other Scissor-like Cutting Tools

A variety of bone cutters are essentially scissors for specialized purposes. Because of the resistance that bone offers to cutting, with these instruments a palmed grip, sometimes with two hands, is needed instead of the finger grip used with other scissors. The jaws of bone-cutting tools close more or less abruptly under great tension as the bone fragments separate. The tips of the blades, therefore, should be clear of any structure you do not desire to include in the cut. For example, while using rib cutters it is customary to point the shears perpendicular to the chest wall with the open blades beside rather than aimed toward the intercostal bundle. After starting a bite into the bone with rongeurs, kerrisons, or other cutters, all tension directed into the wound is relaxed, so that the instrument will not slip deeper as the bite is completed. Security is thus gained when the only tension on the tissue is between the jaws of the instruments.

SUMMARY

Scissors are excellent instruments for cutting and for blunt dissection. Most scissors are designed for use with the right-handed grip that enables direction control and precision of cuts. The thumb-ring finger grip provides the greatest stability in direction control and applies maximal closing, shear, and torque forces with a natural gripping motion of the right hand.

Pronation to neutral hand positions allow the greatest maneuverability of scissors in all directions. The supinated hand can rotate only toward the prone position and therefore has limited maneuverability.

Scissors can cut flaccid tissue effectively since the tissue is stabilized between the scissor blades. Scissor cutting employs closing force, shear, and torque to effect a precise cut. Push-cutting allows straight cuts along the grain of a sheet of tissue. "Chewing" results in a crushed, jagged wound from tissue trapped between the blades of scissors lacking in shear and torque forces.

While cutting sutures with the scissor tips, look for the knot between the slightly spread blades, rather than underneath the scissors. Use the left hand, the patient's body, or another stable structure as a fulcrum to steady the scissors when making delicate cuts or when cutting sutures held by another person. When cutting a row of sutures, hold the sutures in your left hand so that each one becomes taut as you cut it and so that the cut sutures are held out of the way.

Blunt dissection can be achieved by spreading scissor blades between tissue planes or by using the scissors as a rake or probe. Blind dissection is sometimes useful between tissue planes away from vital structures.

Curved scissors offer greater maneuverability and visibility, whereas straight scissors provide the greatest mechanical advantage when cutting tough, thick tissue.

Chapter 3

The Needle Holder

Inefficient use of the needle holder by surgeons accounts for more wasted time than poor technique with any other instrument. There is greater possibility of time loss since a needle holder is used in series with another tool (the needle), and there is a sequence of several steps in taking a stitch. Other tools are more often used singly, or in parallel with another instrument, in one-step maneuvers. There is opportunity to waste time with each clamping and unclamping of the needle holder, as well as between other steps.

The most common mechanisms of time lost are "stuttering" and "stammering" with the needle holder. Stuttering describes the non-productive repetition of steps needed to be done only once. Stammering describes interruption during a step that could be done with one motion.

Stuttering and stammering in surgery are done
with the needle holder.

Stuttering includes:

1. Any repositioning of the needle's angle, direction, and distance from the point in the jaws of the needle holder after receiving a suture from the scrub nurse.
2. Repeatedly going into and out of a wound without taking a stitch, to reposition the needle's angle, point distance, forehand-backhand direction, or to change the exposure.

Stammering occurs after the needle is started into the tissue. Stammering includes:

1. Multiple pushes nearer the eye of the needle.
2. One or more reapplications of the holder during extraction of the needle from the tissue.
3. Superfluous motions while drawing an appropriate length of suture material through the wound, once a stitch is taken.

Stammering, besides losing time due to redundant maneuvers, may waste further time if the needle rotates to a less accessible position when released by the needle holder during unnecessary repositioning.

Another common mechanism of time loss while suturing is the absence of coordinated team effort between surgeon, his assistants, and scrub nurse; this is discussed in Chapter 10.

Self-discipline, more than skill, is required to use a needle holder efficiently.

Self-discipline is needed to force oneself to do each step in suturing once; get tough with yourself.

Force yourself to:

1. Request a suture after first indicating how the needle is to be placed in the holder; then do not readjust the needle position.
2. Take an appropriate grip of the needle holder once.
3. Pass the free end of the stitch to the assistant with one motion.

4. Put the needle point once on the tissue where you want it to enter.
5. Force the needle through the proper bit of tissue with one rotating motion.
6. Release the needle without changing the grip on the needle holder.
7. Grasp the needle once for extraction.
8. Extract the needle from the tissue with one motion.
9. With the needle holder pull the desired length of suture material through the wound and hold the extracted portion of the suture without changing position until an assistant takes it.
10. Reposition the needle on the holder once for the next stitch.

Sewing with a needle holder is a succession of maneuvers with opportunity to waste time at each step. The greatest hazards to efficiency are stuttering and stammering. These two defects can be corrected by sewing in slow motion while using self-discipline to suppress the desire to restart a step. Time spent in slow motion is usually less than that lost by stuttering and stammering. Greater speed will come as efficiency and accuracy become reflex. You will find immediate reward in both time and precision when you eliminate nonproductive repetition of steps.

Stuttering and stammering with a needle holder can become as comfortable a bad habit to a surgeon as saying "you know" several times in a sentence is to a poor conversationalist.

STEPS IN TAKING A STITCH

There are ten steps in taking a stitch; all are important to skillful performance.

There are ten steps in taking a stitch; don't try to get by with fewer.

Step 1.   Positioning the Needle in the Needle Holder

There are two variables: the angle of the needle in the holder, and the location on the needle grasped by the holder. The angle of the needle can be perpendicular, obtuse, acute, or parallel to the holder axis (Fig. 31). If a needle is placed perpendicular to the needle holder (Fig. 31a), the needle can be driven through tissue by merely rotating the holder on its axis; a manipulation that requires no additional space. If, instead, a needle is placed at an oblique or acute angle to the holder (Fig. 31b), the handles must move through a wide arc to follow the curve of the needle while advancing it through tissue. Unfortunately, in difficult access areas where temptation arises to use a nonperpendicular needle attitude to direct the needle, there is less space to move the needle holder handles through the necessary arc. In most cases, it is easier to maneuver a perpendicular needle to the proper attitude than to struggle maneuvering the handles through a wide arc to drive an obtuse or acute angle needle through the tissue. Few situations exist where there is advantage in placing the needle at an acute or an obtuse angle to the holder. The more expert the surgeon, the less his need for curved needle holders and weird needle positions.

A third attitude of the needle is with the plane of its curve parallel to the handles (Fig. 31c), "hooking the needle." Hooking is very useful down in a deep wound when one must sew layers parallel to the surface. This needle attitude eases positioning of the point and requires only a push or a pull to drive the needle through tissue. Such a maneuver uses very little or no space in handle manipulation, compared to oblique attitudes.

There is great advantage in sewing with the needle perpendicular to the needle holder.

The needle may be grasped near the swage or eye, the midportion, or near the point (Fig. 32). Positioning the holder near the swage or eye allows a greater length of the needle to be inserted through the tissue, with less likelihood that the needle will back out of the tissue when the holder lets go. The more the needle point protrudes after inserting a stitch, the easier it is to regrasp during extraction. If the

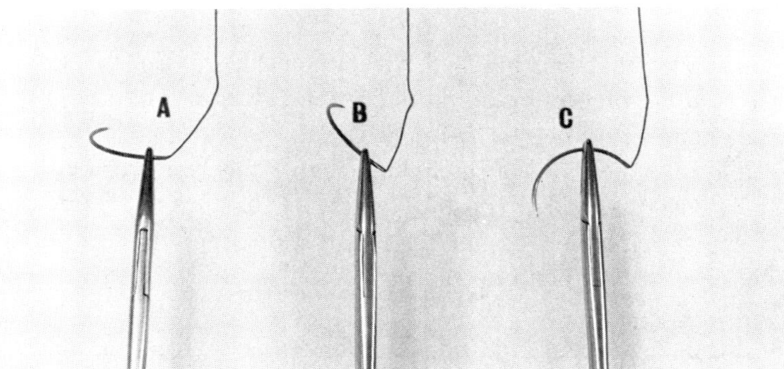

Figure 31. (A) A needle perpendicular to holder is ideally made to perform in limited space by rotating the holder on its axis. (B) With needle at an angle not perpendicular to the holder, space may not permit the wider arc needed to advance the needle through tissue. (C) "Hooking the needle," where the plane of the needle curve is parallel to the handles, is useful in deep wound sewing of layers parallel to the surface.

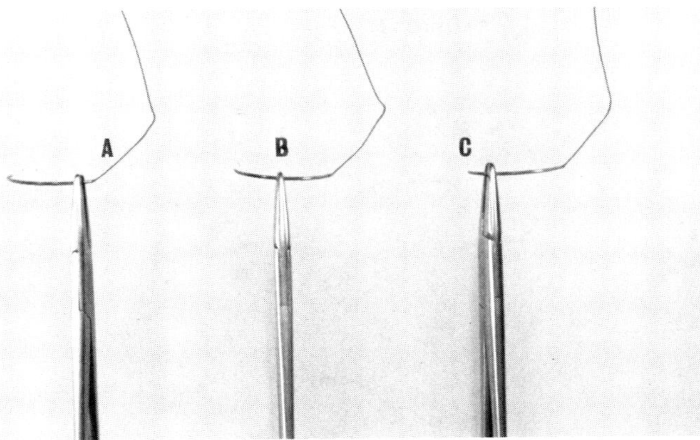

Figure 32. (A) Grasping the needle near the eye works best for soft tissue. It allows maximum needle length to be inserted through tissue, least risk of needle slippage, and maximum exposure of point for regrasping. (B) When the needle is grasped near midpoint, rather than near the eye, greater force is available to advance the needle through tissue, with less risk of breakage. (C) For tough tissue, the needle is grasped near the point, for greatest driving force. As the needle is advanced, the holder is repositioned nearer to the eye.

needle is clamped too near or on the swage or eye, breakage is common.

The closer to the point the needle is grasped, the greater the driving force that can be used without breakage. So, for soft tissue, there is advantage in grasping nearer the swage or eye, and in tough tissue, nearer the point. In tough tissue, as the needle is advanced, multiple reapplications of the holder nearer the swage or eye are occasionally essential and purposeful, and are therefore not "stammering." The same principles of needle application apply whether using a forehand or a backhand needle position.

Step 2. Grasping the Needle Holder Each of four needle holder grips (Figs. 33–36) has mechanical advantage and disadvantage, which should dictate its use in specific situations.

There are advantages and disadvantages to all needle holder grips.

THE PALMED GRIP. As shown in Figure 33, this is the strongest grip and therefore provides the greatest pressure in driving

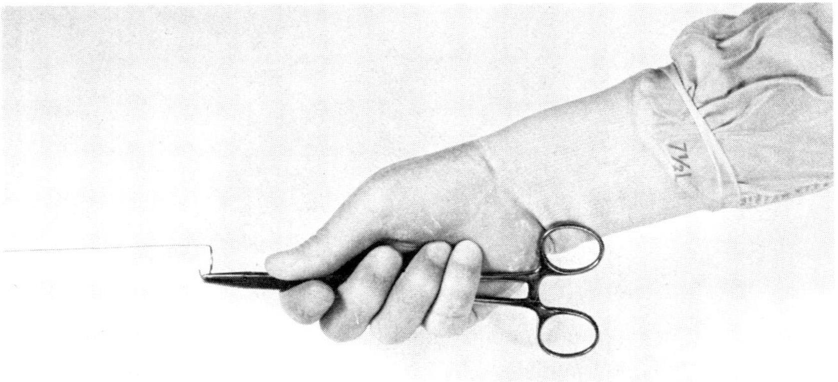

Figure 33. The palmed grip of the holder affords greatest pressure and control of needle in tough tissue. The drawback is the need to change the grip to release or regrasp the needle.

a needle through tough material such as thick scar, cartilage, and bone. Another advantage of this grip is that the thumb and index finger grasp the holder near the needle, thereby giving maximal control of needle movement. With the palmed grip, the needle holder can be rotated in the palm between the fingers and thumb for any desired direction of the needle point. This opportunity for manipulation allows pronation to begin a stitch and supination to extract a needle, unlimited by the range of motion of the hand and arm; the thumb grip (Fig. 35) is subject to this limitation.

A disadvantage of the palmed grip is that the needle cannot be released and regrasped after a stitch is taken without readjusting to another grip. Changing a grip in the middle of a stitch always moves and stresses the tissue in the needle bite, and may dislodge the needle. This stress and movement may be acceptable with tough material, but is unacceptable with fragile structures where tears might result.

Another disadvantage is that use of the left hand may be necessary during the release to stabilize the instrument while shifting from palmed grip to another. Such a maneuver interrupts whatever exposure or other function was being provided by the left hand. Special needle holders, such as the Castroviejo, have locking devices that will release with the squeeze of the hand, thereby minimizing the disadvantages of the palmed grip during delicate work. In general, the palmed needle grip is most advantageous when strong needle driving force is required to sew tough tissue.

THE THENAR GRIP. The needle holder may be grasped between the ball of the thumb and either the ring finger or little finger (Fig. 34). The greatest advantage of the thenar grip is time saved during continuous suturing, by elimination of steps of other methods. The needle can be released and regrasped for extraction without changing grips, as is necessary with the palmed position. The needle can be redirected in preparation for the next stitch by spinning the holder clockwise in the palm without the need for readjusting the needle in the holder or changing grips, as is necessary with the "thumb grip."

The thenar grip allows as much mobility in supination as the palmed grip and rates between the thumb–ring finger grip and the pencil grip in both strength and direction control. The disadvantage of the thenar grip is lack of precision when releasing the needle. When

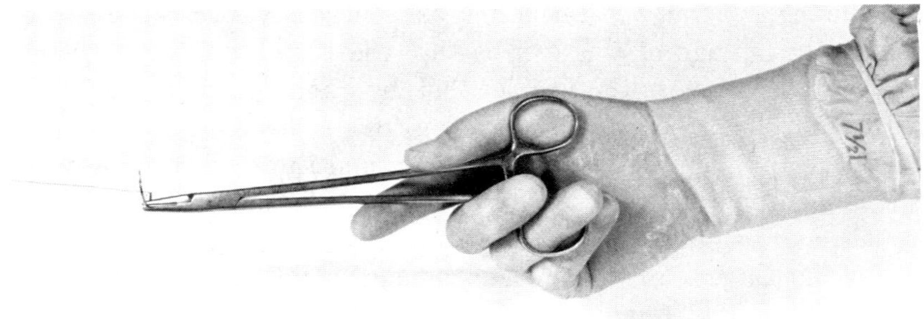

Figure 34. The thenar grip, with ball of thumb on shaft of needle holder and with ring finger or little finger in finger ring, allows release and regrasp of needle, as well as redirection of needle. The "popping" release risks unplanned needle movement.

a needle holder is locked, there is spring tension between the handles. To unlock, thenar eminence pressure is exerted perpendicular to the shafts until the teeth of the lock are suddenly distracted. The spring tension then pops the handles apart. It is difficult to prevent some movement of the needle at that time.

The "thenar grip" is a versatile method of grasping the needle holder, but is an affectation when using other surgical tools.

THE THUMB–RING FINGER GRIP. The greatest advantage of the thumb–ring finger grip (Fig. 35) is that it allows precision when releasing a needle. With the thumb and ring finger in the finger rings, the needle can be released without stressing the tissue by inadvertent motion of the needle holder. By exerting closing pressure between the thumb and ring finger, spring tension of the handles can be relieved from the lock before distracting the teeth. The needle can then be released without the characteristic "pop" of the thenar grip release. Regrasping to extract a needle is also precise with the thumb grip, as a greater range of motion is well controlled with the digits in the two finger rings.

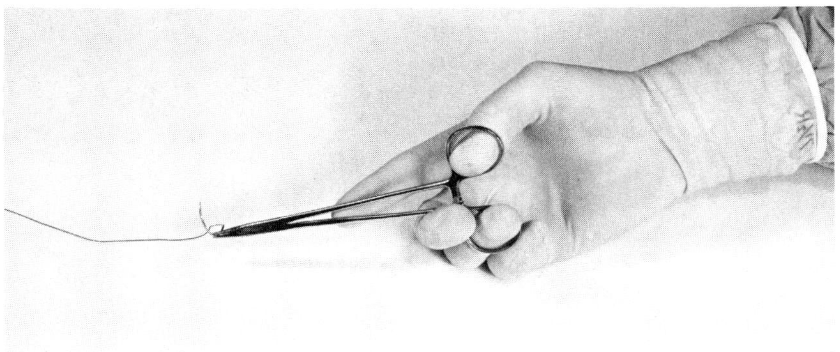

Figure 35. The thumb and ring finger grip, with these digits controlling the needle holder from the finger rings, is suited to delicate work; needle release is achieved without undue tissue stress, and regrasping is precise.

In delicate work, such as small blood vessel suturing, the release and, occasionally, the regrasp of the needle are the most critical steps. During these steps fragile tissue is easily torn. In critically important stitches, the more precise thumb–ring finger grip is a better alternative than a more rapid method.

It may be better to be precise than rapid.

PENCIL GRIP. The pencil grip is the most delicate and accurate method for very fine suturing. This grip is best used with spring opening needle holders with finger pressure release locks or no locks at all. The Castroviejo needle holder (Fig. 36) is an example. The pencil grip allows the needle to be driven through tissue by rotating the holder on its axis between the index finger and thumb. This grip is applicable to eye surgery as well as to fine vascular and nerve work, because needle control is provided with fine movements of the fingers.

Left-hand support of the needle holder is occasionally useful to increase control while sewing with any of the grips.

Because of the advantages of each grip in specific application, skill should be developed in using each.

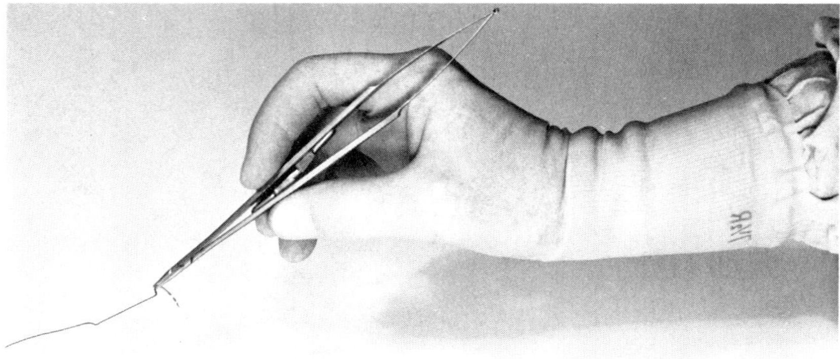

Figure 36. The pencil grip is shown with the Castroviejo needle holder, with finger pressure release lock. Index finger and thumb can control precise movements for very fine suturing.

Step 3. Positioning the Free End of the Suture

This is the most frequently forgotten step. Before putting the needle into the wound, pass the free end of the suture to the assistant's side of the field (Figs. 33–36). This step has two benefits: The assistant can prevent tangling of the free end in other sutures or clamps and can begin knot tying without having to fumble for the free end after a stitch is taken. This step is most frequently eliminated or forgotten at the most critical stitches deep in a hole, the one place where it is most important to prevent tangling and make the most of assistants. The more critical the stitch, the more important it is to include each step. Shortcuts may be useful during easy work, but they make difficult maneuvers even more so. Don't hide the free end from your helpers (Fig. 37).

If there are more steps in inserting a stitch than you think, you are probably leaving out the most important one.

Don't hide the free end of a suture from the assistant and then expect help.

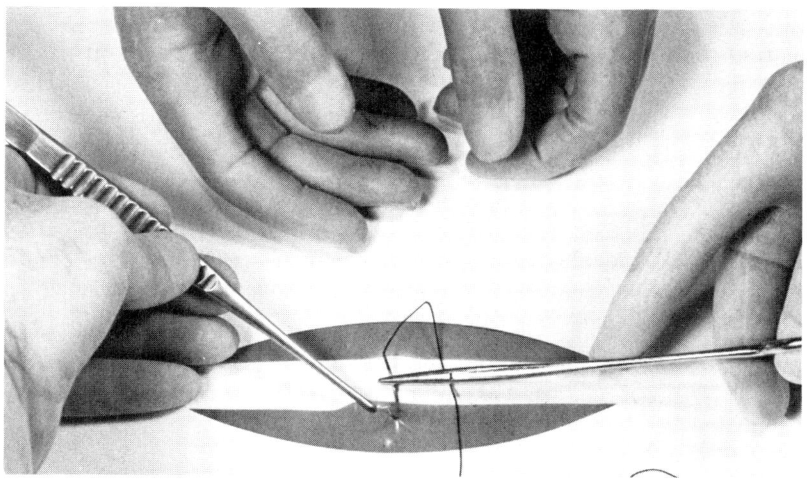

Figure 37. To insure against tangling and to allow for prompt knot tying, pass the free suture end to the assistant's side before stitching.

Step 4. Placement of the Needle Point

The fourth step is to place the needle point at the proper site with the body attitude necessary to take the desired bite of tissue. In an awkward spot it takes more self-discipline during this step than in any other; here "stuttering" is most likely to occur. As you start into a wound with a needle, resolve to yourself: "I am going to put the needle point where I want it the first time, no matter what." Strangely, such discipline will account for better needle positioning than that given by many indecisive needle readjustments.

Hand position and direction of approach are important factors in gaining optimal mechanical advantage for placing the needle to take a stitch. A forehand stitch is done with a supinating motion. Therefore, starting with the hand in pronation gives 180° maneuverability to rotate the needle through the tissue. Conversely, to place such a stitch starting with the palm up, the only way to obtain further supination following the curve of the needle is to raise the surgeon off the floor and rotate him toward the left by pressure from his elbow against his side.

It is bad manners for the elbow to push the surgeon away from the operative field. There is no advantage to sewing with your shoulder in your ear, your foot off the floor, and your spine in scoliosis. If your elbow is touching your side, something needs to be turned 180°.

In taking a forehand stitch, optimal mechanical advantage ensues when approaching the tissue from the opposite side—sewing toward oneself (Fig. 38). To sew away from oneself in a forehand manner presses the elbow against the ribs, the shoulder against the ear, the left foot off the floor, and the spine in scoliosis, and in general, forces the surgeon away from the operative field (Fig. 39).

Forehand sewing introduces the needle toward oneself; backhand sewing introduces the needle away from oneself.

Conversely, when suturing backhand, starting with the palms up and sewing away from oneself gives optimal maneuverability and mechanical advantage.

Step 5. *Putting the Needle Through the Tissue*

With a curved needle there are two force vectors that need to be balanced to give minimal stress on the wound: (a) driving force that pushes the needle through the tissue (Fig. 40D); and (b) rotating force that keeps the proper needle curve attitude in the tissue (Fig. 40R). A half-circle needle needs to be rotated 180° as it is forced through its course. If rotation is less than 180°, the swage or eye will tend to lacerate tissue toward the concavity of the needle, commonly referred to as "not following the curve of the needle." Conversely, a rotation of greater than 180°, "torquing the needle," will tend to lacerate with the swage or eye on the convex aspect of the needle.

The driving force is in the direction of the segment of needle within the tissue. The driving force does not rotate with the curve of

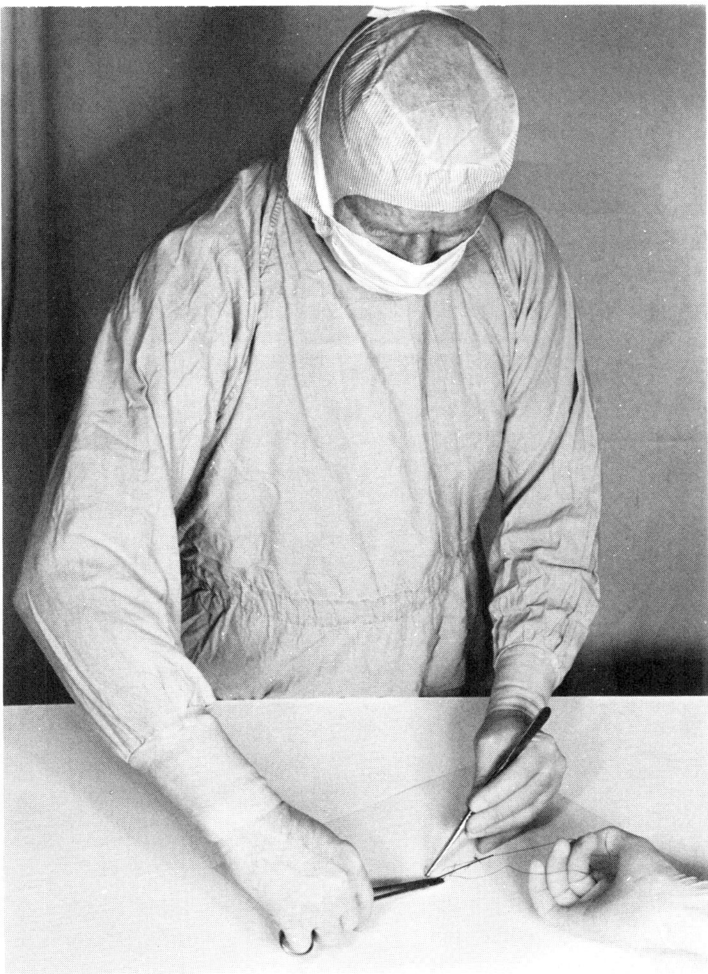

Figure 38. Optimal method for a forehand stitch is to start with prone hand and sew toward oneself, affording full 180° scope to rotate needle through tissue.

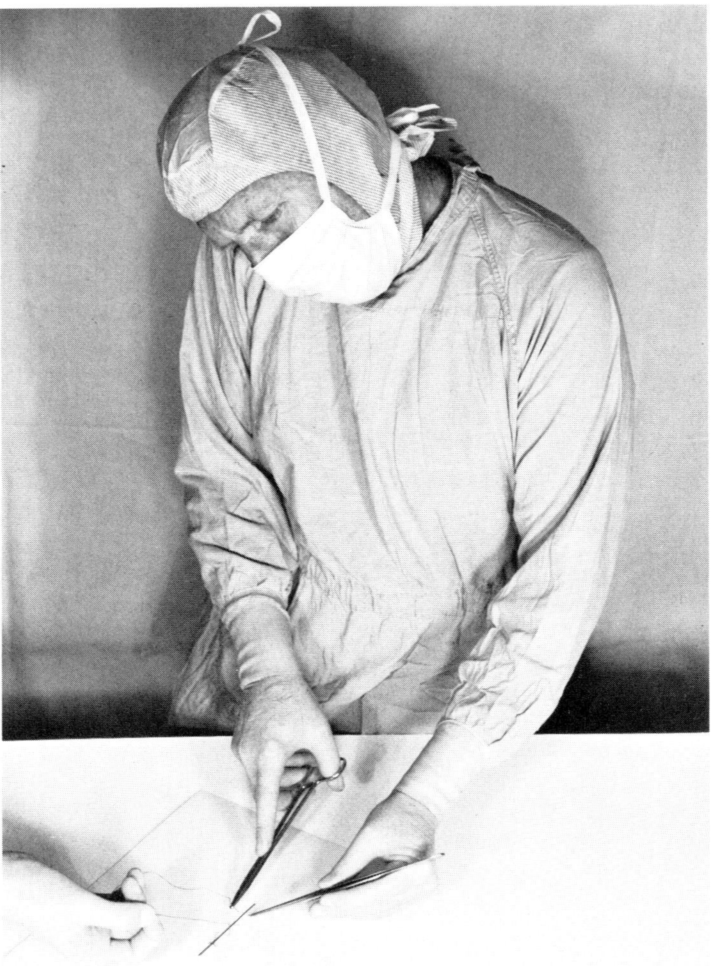

Figure 39. Sewing away from oneself to take a forehand stitch forces a cramped, counterproductive body attitude.

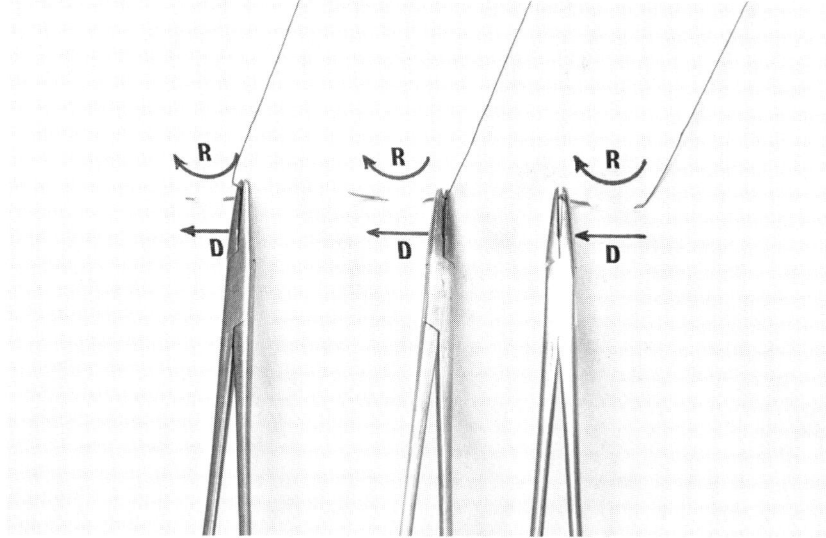

Figure 40. The driving force (D) is always in the direction of the segment of needle within the tissue. The rotating force (R) maintains nonstressed attitude of the needle in the tissue.

the needle; it has the same direction no matter whether the point, shaft, or eye is within the tissue (Fig. 40). In other words, the tissue segment of the needle stays in the same direction even though the needle is rotated during its course. Therefore, the drive force is not in the direction of the point of the needle except at the beginning of the stitch.

"Follow the curve of the needle" may be an ambiguous instruction to one who doesn't understand both force vectors of curved needle driving.

If the needle is advanced in the tissue to its holder junction with as much needle point showing as possible, extraction is facilitated. A needle barely showing its point may back out when released, so that the point disappears into the tissue, requiring redriving or retaking of the stitch.

When sewing tough tissue, cartilage, or scar tissue, steady sustained mild pressure will advance the needle where greater force will merely break the needle.

Step 6. Needle Release

Before releasing a needle, one of two alternatives of needle support can prevent dislodgment or change in the needle attitude between release and the regrasping for extraction. Tissue forceps can grasp the needle point or support the tissue on the needle, stabilizing for reapplication of the holder to the exposed joint. Where tissue is very fragile and the attiude of the needle point is unlikely to change after being released, support may be contraindicated; tissue may be torn if the needle is held by two nonsynchronous instruments. Accurate releasing of a needle without stressing the tissue is the most critical step of suturing, and the most difficult to master.

Releasing the needle is the most critical and difficult step
in suturing.

Step 7. Regrasping the Needle for Extraction

Make an effort to grasp the needle perpendicular to the holder, to simplify the rotation vector force for easy nontraumatic completion of the stitch. The more critical the stitch, the greater the advantage of perpendicular regrasp of the needle.

Step 8. Needle Extraction

The same principles of following the curve of the needle and the proper force vectors discussed under Step 5 apply to needle extraction. Take care to continue proper rotation force and proper driving force in the direction of the needle segment in the tissue.

Two alternative hand positions, pronation or supination, can be used in needle extraction. Grasping the needle with the hand pronated allows 180° supinating motion of the hand to follow the curve of the needle. This position gives the greatest security against tearing the swage or eye of the needle through delicate tissue. Pronation at the beginning of extraction leaves the hand and body uncramped and in a functional position.

The supinated grasp of a needle for extraction has the advantage, in some cases, of saving time. If the needle has been inserted far enough so that it can be grasped away from the point, near the center, regrasping with the hand in supination allows the next stitch to be taken without readjustment of the needle in the holder. The time saved may be imaginary if the needle insertion for the succeeding stitch requires an additional step of reapplication of the holder during the driving of the needle through the tissue in order to advance the point far enough for the next extraction. The great disadvantage is that a supinated hand cannot be supinated more without twisting the body with the elbow against the side, the shoulder in the ear, and the left foot off the floor. Imprecision, the hazard of tearing tissue, and the awkward position make the timesaving value suspect.

Don't sacrifice accuracy and safety in the patient to save the time of a maneuver out in the room.

Step 9. Pulling the Desired Length of Suture Through the Wound

During interrupted suturing, if Step 3 has not been forgotten, the assistant can establish the desired length by holding the free end the distance from the wound that will give him the optimal length for tying. If continuous suturing is done, the surgeon pulls the stitch until he has established the desired amount of tension on the suture line, then allows time for transfer of that tension to the assistant. In both cases, the surgeon holds the needle end in an accessible position until the assistant has control of it.

Dropping the needle end before the assistant has control may cause lost time from entanglement with other sutures or clamps, and loss of uniform tension on the wound. Wasted excess motions can be prevented by pulling the desired length of suture with one uninterrupted motion with the needle holder after grasping the needle for extraction. Hand-over-hand pulling of a suture through the wound is "stammering."

Step 10. Reposition the Needle on the Holder for the Next Stitch

During interrupted suturing it takes no additional time to reposition the needle on the holder before handing it to the scrub nurse, as it is done while the assistant is tying and the surgeon is otherwise unoccupied. By placing the needle in the holder exactly as desired for the next stitch, and placing the handle toward the scrub nurse, the surgeon not only guarantees proper needle placement but eliminates the step of needle readjustment by an instrument nurse. If an assistant is following the suture, reversing Steps 9 and 10, repositioning the needle before pulling through the suture, divides the extraction motion into two motions without any advantage.

When you help the assistant and instrument nurse you may be helping yourself and the patient.

When approximating two sides of a wound with sutures, time can be saved by picking up both sides with the same bite of the needle, provided the needle is long enough to allow easy grasping of the point for extraction. Better alignment of wound ends is accomplished, however, if the stitches at each end of the wound are taken with separate bites on each side.

STRAIGHT NEEDLES

Hand-held straight needles, such as Keiths, eliminate the need of a needle holder and therefore are simpler, faster and more precise in some applications. Hand-held needles, unlike those used with needle holder, do not require two hands to reposition the needle for the next stitch. A straight needle gives better opportunity to direct its point without bending or breaking, once the tissue has been entered. On the other hand, a curved needle's course is essentially predetermined by the shape of the curve as soon as the needle enters the tissue. A straight needle can never change its attitude to an inaccessible one by turning, as can occur when a curved needle slips in a needle holder's grasp. Furthermore, after inserting a hand-held needle it is not necessary to let go completely to regrasp it for exraction. The straight needle, held between the thumb, index, and middle fingers as it enters the tissue (Fig. 41), can be regrasped by the thumb and index finger near the point, while still maintaining pressure and control of the swage end with the side of the ring finger (Fig. 42). The tip of the ring finger thus acts much like the thimble-covered fingertip of a needleworker. Inserting, extracting, and readying the needle for the next stitch thus becomes one continuous, efficient movement of the right hand, with the left hand free for other manipulations. The major disadvantage of straight needles is that they cannot be used in a depression. They are therefore useful only on convex surfaces (e.g., skin) and other organs that can be delivered out of the wound (e.g., small bowel).

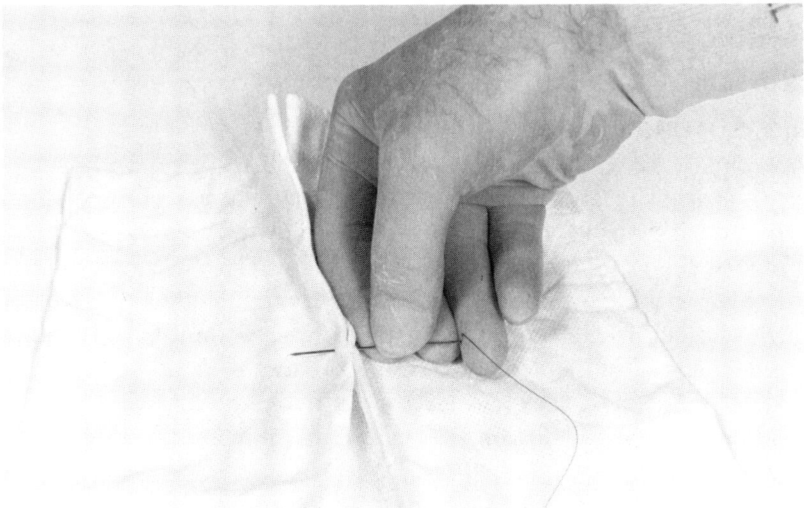

Figure 41. As it is inserted, the hand-held straight needle is grasped by thumb, index, and middle fingers.

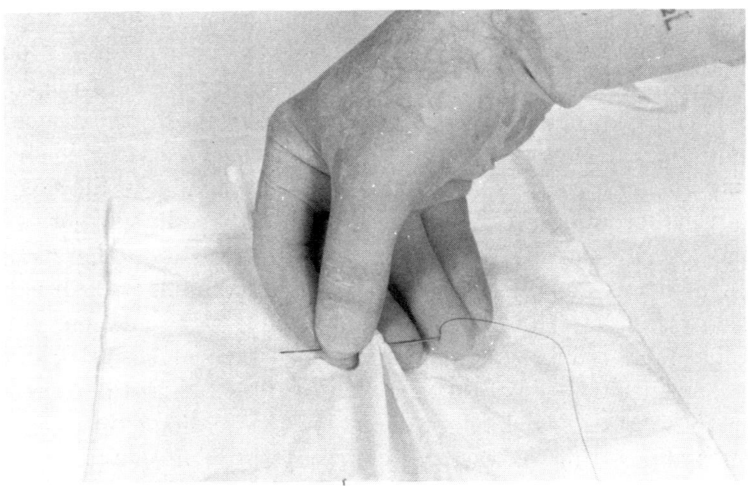

Figure 42. The straight needle is extracted by regrasping near the point with thumb and index finger, bracing the swage end with the side of the ring finger.

If two methods are equally safe, the simpler one is the better.

WIRE SUTURES USING AN AWL

A Rochester awl may be used to put wire sutures through bone, such as during closure of a sternal-splitting incision. Using the thumb and index finger as a depth stop, and drilling or rotating the needle alternately clockwise and counterclockwise with minimal pressure, the needle can be inserted to a precise depth without any hazard of slipping deeper than intended. Extracting the awl with wire attached is also facilitated by a back-and-forth rotation of the instrument. Such motion requires less traction than needed with a steady pull.

FOLLOWING THE SUTURE

The suture follower can accomplish three objectives:

1. He can maintain proper tension on the suture line.
2. He can keep the redundant suture material out of the way of the operator.
3. He can help expose the operative field for the next stitch.

The surgeon should pull through a continuous suture to the tension he desires, then pass it to the assistant. If the assistant grasps the suture halfway between the needle and the wound (Fig. 43), he can then maintain tension on the suture line, while eliminating excessive redundant suture material that would be in the way of the operator. Increased suture length toward the needle to allow manipulation of the needle by the operator can be made by supinating the hand, whereas excess slack which would get in the operator's way can be taken up by pronating the hand. The supination and pronation to leave the required redundant length toward the needle can be adjusted while still maintaining tension on the previous stitch. Tension maintained on the suture line by the assistant will tent up the layer being sutured and

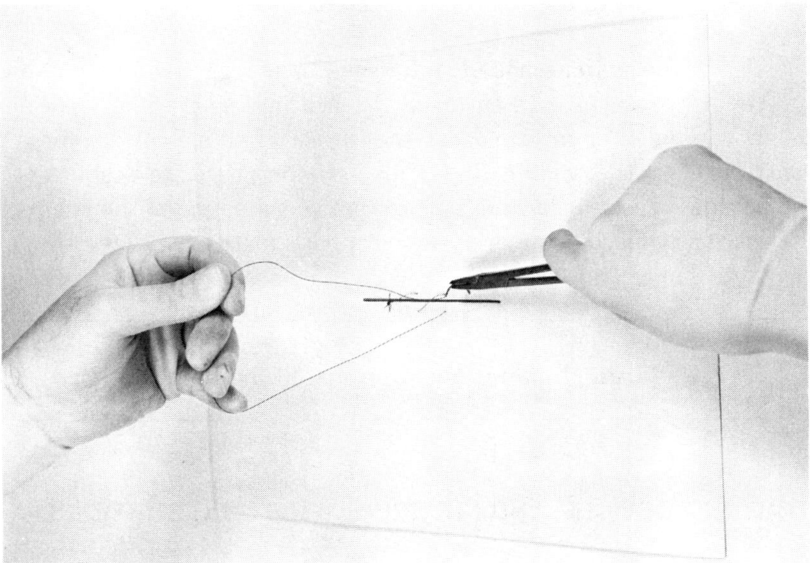

Figure 43. When the assistant grasps the suture halfway between the needle and the wound, he can adjust both tension and redundant length by supinating or pronating his hand.

thereby expose the field for the succeeding stitch. After a stitch is taken, the suture is released by the assistant just before tension is applied to the redundant loop by the surgeon. Coordination is required to prevent the loss of tension on the suture line by too early a release by the assistant.

It takes two to tango, but only one to tangle.

The suture follower can facilitate efficiency when lock stitches are used if he holds the suture toward the direction of the needle in such a way that the sewing is done within the redundant loop, thus requiring no extra motion for locking. Mattress suturing can be facilitated if the operator pulls the suture through the wound on the alternate bite that goes towards the assistant. The suture can then be followed without the assistant's being in the operator's way. If the deep stitch is being placed toward the assistant, that is the one that is pulled through and held. Pulling alternate sutures precludes the need for the assistant to hold the redundant suture on alternating sides of the suture line.

In some situations, it is advantageous for a surgeon to follow his own suture. An example is in suturing the beating heart, where the left thumb and index finger can grasp the suture a half inch away from the heart, placing the middle finger against the tissue to stabilize the wound, and sense cardiac motions so that coordination of the needle to the heartbeat becomes merely a coordinate motion between the left and right hands.

Dysdiadochokinesia is a poor trait in a surgeon.

STAPLING DEVICES AND FUTURE SOPHISTICATED TOOLS

Stapling devices and future sophisticated tools should replace or supplement older utensils whenever they do a superior job. Older surgeons need to guard against sticking to old tools out of prejudice and inertia. Stapling devices offer real advantages in many applications. Besides saving time, the simultaneous closure of the whole width of a suture line, with uniform tension and without intermittent distortion and trauma due to the stress of individual suture points, may be of clinical value. A further advantage of stapling devices is the hemostasis without interstitial hematomas produced by cutting vessels, then clamping, and ligating. It is well to realize that disadvantages pointed out by surgeons who have no facility or little experience in the use of a tool may represent deficiencies in their method of application, rather than disadvantages of the tool itself. Enumeration of the disadvantages of a tool or method by one who has not used it may be a mere exercise in self-deception.

Old dogs need to learn new tricks.

SUMMARY

Suturing efficiently requires orderly performing of each of ten steps, without omission. Each step should be done with self-discipline, to prevent stuttering and stammering. Sewing can be made awkward by starting a motion requiring supination with the hand already in full supination, i.e., forehand sewing away from oneself. Follow this clue to prevent awkward sewing attitudes: if the elbow touches the side, it is time to change something 180°.

Chapter 4

Tissue Forceps

Tissue forceps are nonlocking, grasping tools. They can be used with the left hand to assist maneuvers with the right. Tissue forceps, therefore, are almost in constant use as an adjunct to the needle holder, scalpel, scissors, clamp, or whatever other tool is being used by the right hand. Extensive practice to develop facility with this most-used instrument will be time well spent.

How To Hold Tissue Forceps

Hold the tissue forceps so that one blade functions as an extension of the thumb, and the other blade as an extension of the opposing fingers. Grasp with the forceps, using the same motion as grasping with the empty hand (Fig. 44). The pencil position or the position shown in Figure 44, with the shanks against the index finger metacarpal-phalangeal joint, gives the widest range of maneuverability with the forceps. Holding the shank in the palm as shown in Figure 45, has little, if any, use in surgery; the tips can only gain access to a wound by extreme flexion of the wrist, thereby severely limiting the range of useful motion of the forceps.

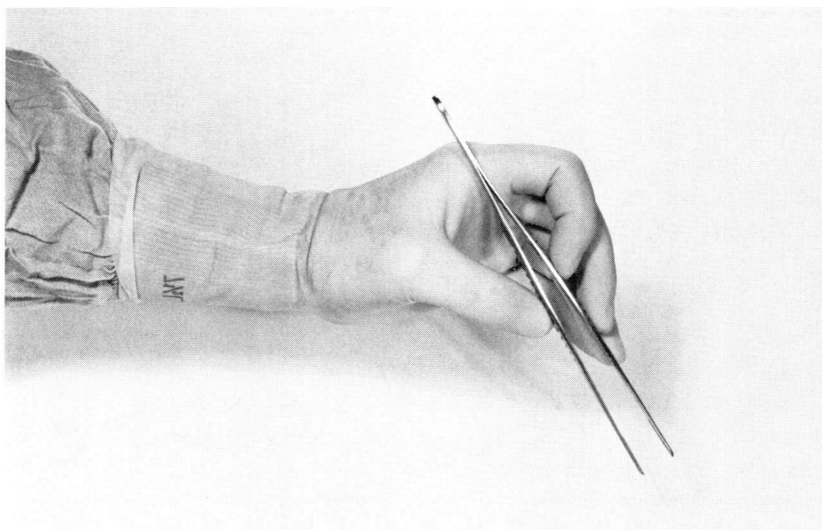

Figure 44. The modified pencil-like grasp of tissue forceps is, with one blade an extension of the thumb, and the other blade an extension of the opposing fingers.

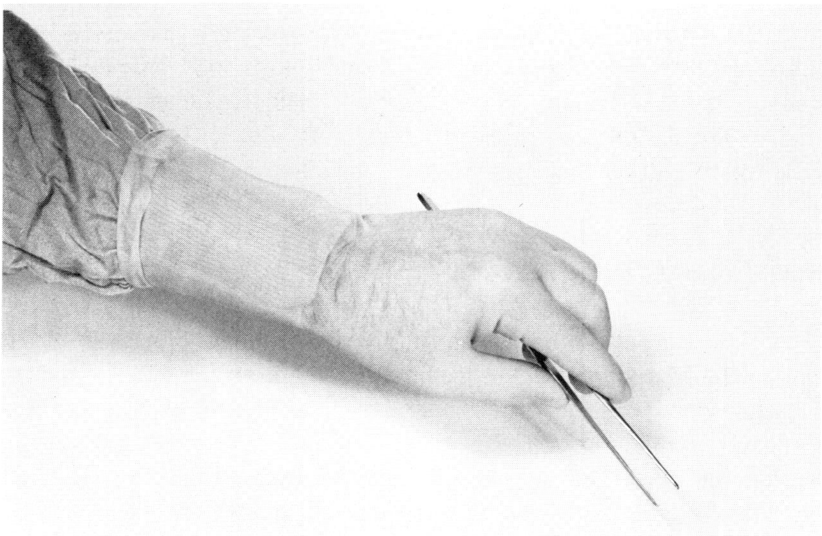

Figure 45. The palm grip of forceps requires too great a wrist flexion to gain access to a wound.

A palm grip of the forceps can be useful only for sewing on the ceiling.

Holding Forceps Not in Use

When alternately needing to grasp with forceps and fingers, as when sewing then tying sutures, palming the forceps, as in Figure 46, can save time lost from repeatedly discarding and retrieving them. Holding the forceps with the ring and little fingers, with the distal interphalangeal joints in extension (Fig. 46) frees the middle finger to maneuver through a wider range of motion than when the forceps are grasped by flexed phalanges (Fig. 47). The flexor digitorum profundus muscle has a common muscle belly to the middle, ring, and little fingers, so flexion of the distal joints of two fingers to hold the forceps also flexes the middle finger. Having the distal joints of the ring and

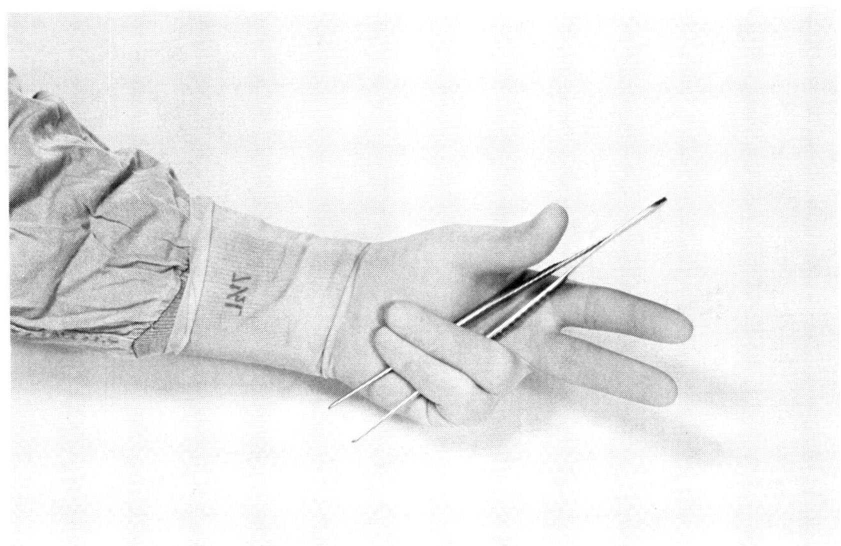

Figure 46. When not in active use, forceps may be palmed and supported by *extended* ring finger and little finger, leaving a useful *unflexed* middle finger.

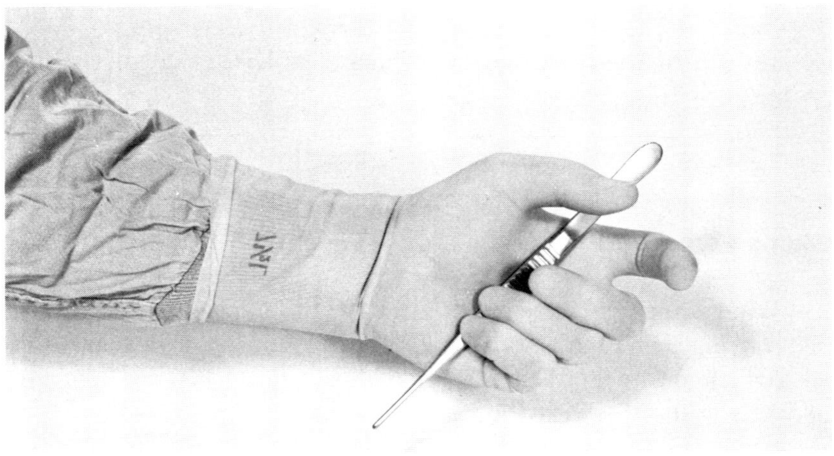

Figure 47. Supporting the palmed forceps by flexed ring finger and little finger removes from service the automatically flexed middle finger.

little finger in extension when grasping the forceps leaves the flexor digitorum profundus muscle relaxed, making possible full, free extension of the middle finger for other manipulation. When left-hand little finger and ring finger manipulation is needed during a portion of one-handed tying, temporarily shift the palmed forceps to a pinch in the web between the thumb and index finger.

The flexor digitorum profundus sends tendons to the distal phalanges of the long, ring, and small digits, so flexion of the distal interphalangeal joints of two fingers also flexes the third.

Changing Forceps from "Hold" to "Use" Position

Changing from "hold" to a "use" position can be done with one motion without climbing up and down the forceps, if they are first grasped at the proper spot with the thumb and index finger. The proper grasp is difficult with the palm up, as gravity causes the forceps to lie against the palm, requiring extreme metacarpal-phalangeal joint flexion of the thumb and index finger (Figs. 48 and 49).

Grasping at the proper spot is made easier by turning the palm down (Fig. 50), so that gravity moves the forceps away from the palm; the index finger and thumb can then grasp the desired place without extreme flexion of their metacarpal-phalangeal joints.

Smooth and efficient transfer of the forceps from the "use" to the "hold" position and back again becomes automatic, secure, and comfortable with practice.

Bad habits are always more comfortable than newly tried, superior methods.

Tissue Forceps Approach to a Wound

There is maximum mobility in the use of tissue forceps if the wound is approached from opposite sides by the two hands. If your left and right hand approach the wound from the same side or end, your

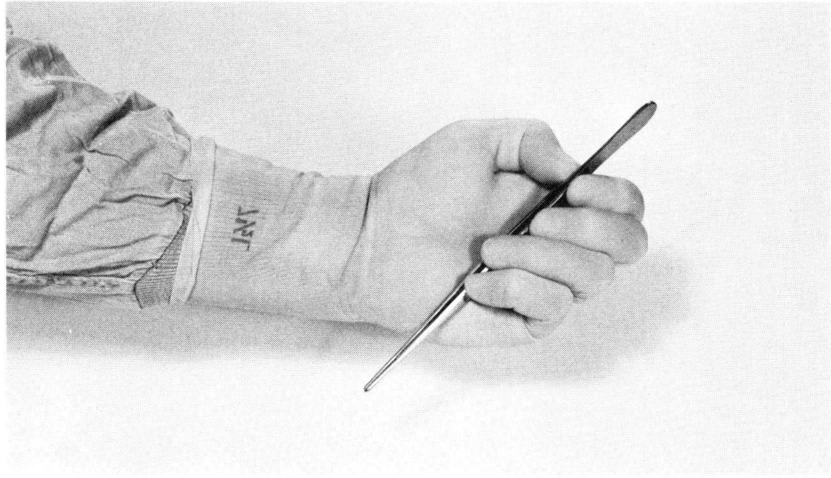

Figure 48. To change from "hold" to "use" position, with the palm up, gravity makes the grasp too far from the tips.

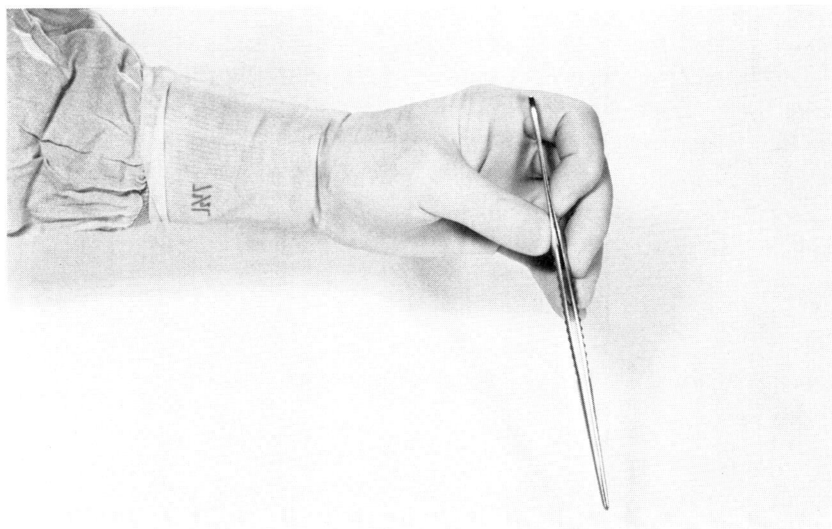

Figure 49. Shift from a hold position too far from the tips requires an additional adjustment.

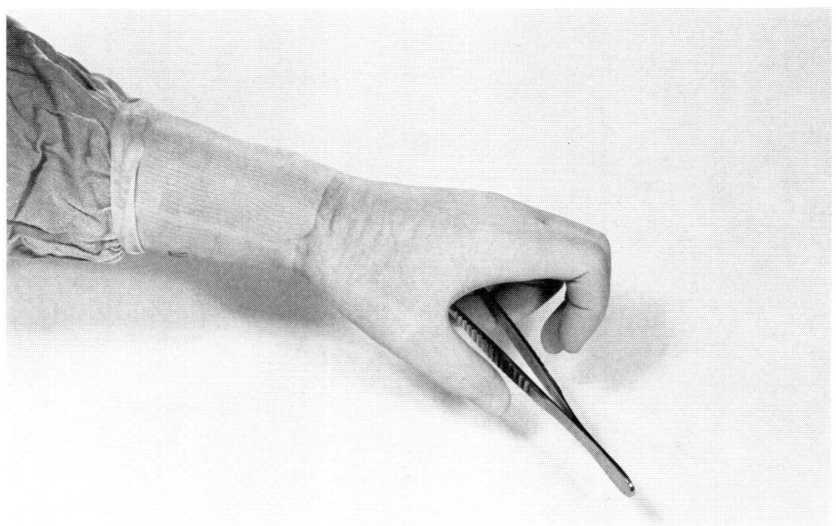

Figure 50. With palm down, gravity aids the desired shift from hold to use position of forceps.

two elbows will lie close to the sides of your body, limiting the mobility of both extremities (Fig. 51). Any movement of the body to the left, to free the right hand, further cramps the left. Also, any motion of the body to the right, to free the left hand, in the same way compromises the ability of the right.

When approaching the wound with left and right hands from opposite sides, turning the body can always free an elbow from the side, increasing mobility of one extremity without cramping the other hand (Fig. 52). There is, therefore, advantage in mobility by approaching the wound with the forceps from the side or end *opposite* to the instrument in the right hand.

To improve mobility, forceps maneuvers requiring wrist flexion should be started in wrist extension, and vice versa. Maneuvers that require supination should be started in pronation, and vice versa.

Maneuvers requiring pronation should be started in supination, and vice versa.

Forceps Uses

Forceps are used to hold tissue during cutting; retract for exposure; stabilize during suturing; extract needles; grasp vessels for cautery; pass ligatures around hemostats deep in wound; pack sponges; grasp free objects for extraction; and clear blood with cottonoid or other small sponges.

Where To Grasp

When sewing, particularly on the skin, visualize the point where the stitch is to enter before grasping the tissue with the forceps. Grasping can distort and give false perspective, thereby resulting in inproperly lined up closure. Grasp the tissue away from the point of needle entrance. A common error of the beginner is to hold the tissue at the desired point of needle entrance, thereby blocking that point and

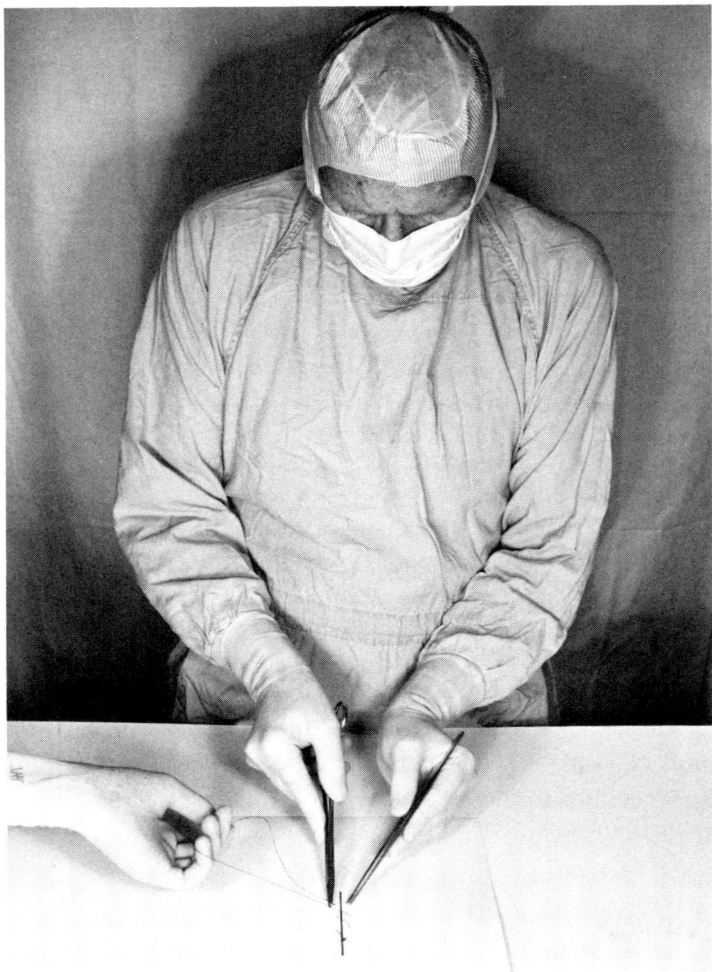

Figure 51. Tissue forceps approach to the wound that forces elbows close to the body unduly restricts mobility.

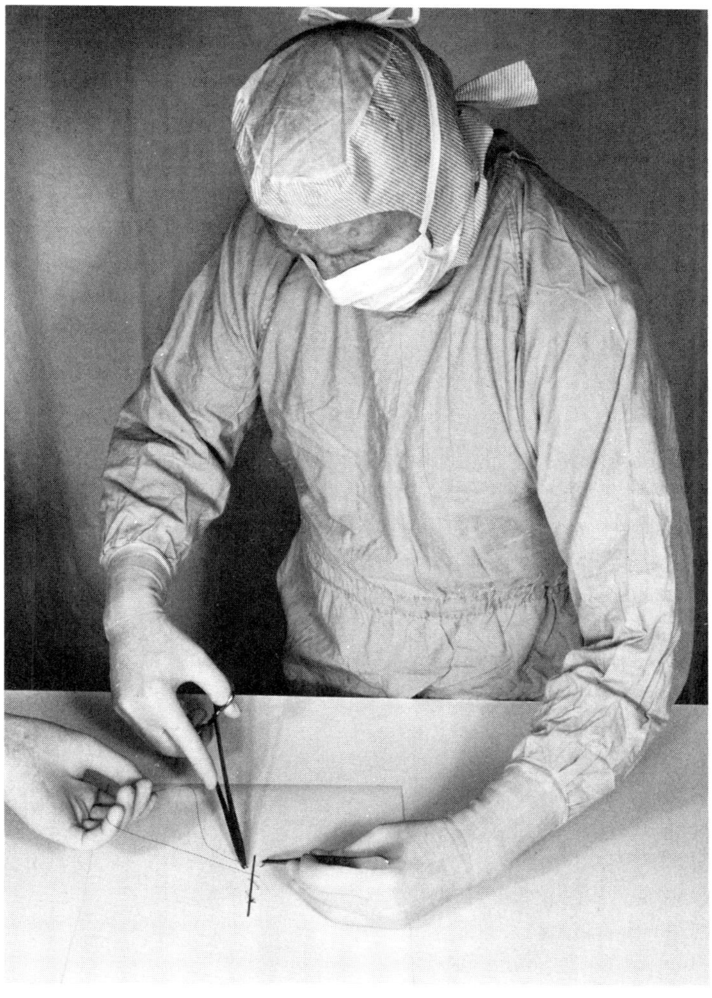

Figure 52. With elbows wide, both hands are afforded maximum maneuverability.

forcing a different bite. Instead, the tissue forceps should be used to expose and stabilize comfortably away from the site of needle entrance.

Don't use your forceps to block your needle.

During suturing, the usefulness of the tissue forceps can be expanded from merely picking up the layer to be sutured, to include increasing accuracy and exposure, if the following four positions are used with each stitch.

Step 1.

On the far side of the wound, grasp the layer above the one to be sutured and retract upward and outward with the tissue forceps, thereby widely exposing the layer to be sutured (Fig. 53). The needle point is then placed at the desired level.

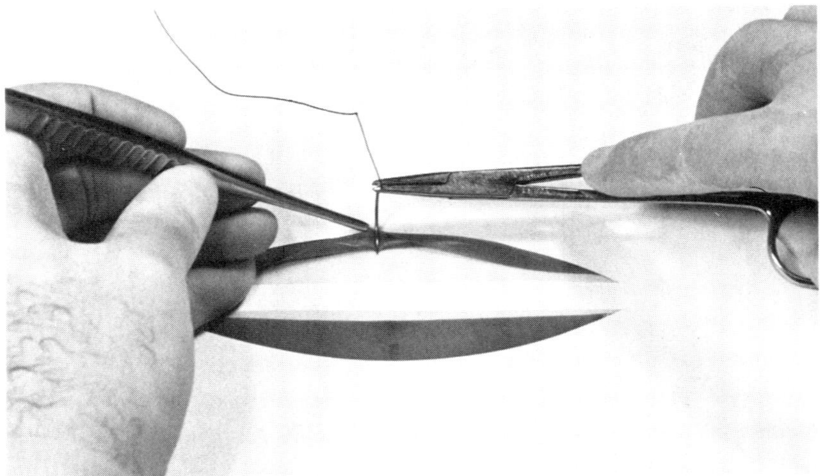

Figure 53. In suturing, Step 1 use of forceps is increasing exposure by retracting the far-side layer above the one to be stitched.

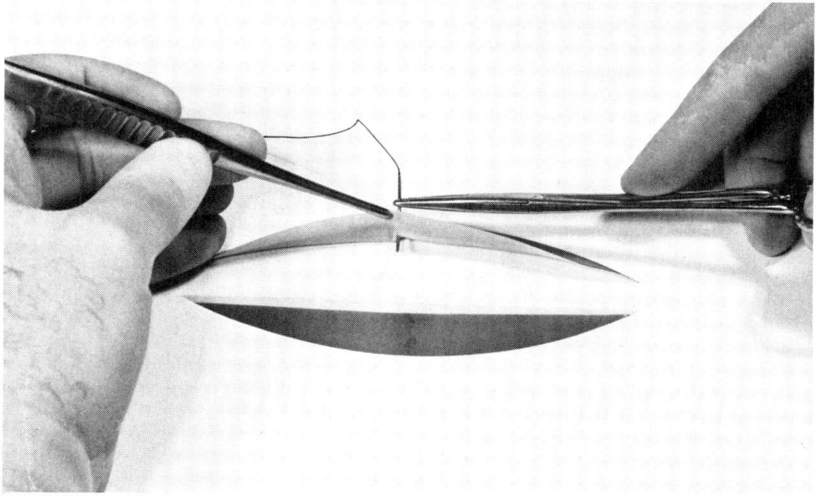

Figure 54. After needle entry, Step 2 use of forceps is lifting the far-side layer being sutured to expose needle exit.

Step 2.

Before driving the needle completely through the tissue, move the forceps from the superficial layer and grasp the layer being sutured. Then lift to expose the needle exit as it is driven through the tissue (Fig. 54).

Step 3.

On the near side of the wound grasp the layer being sewed and lift to expose the desired needle entrance site (Fig. 55).

Step 4.

After placing the needle point at the desired site, move the tissue forceps and retract the more superficial layer, thereby exposing the needle exit site (Fig. 56).

By moving the tissue forceps from superficial to deep layer on the far side, and from the deep to the superficial layer on the near side, the

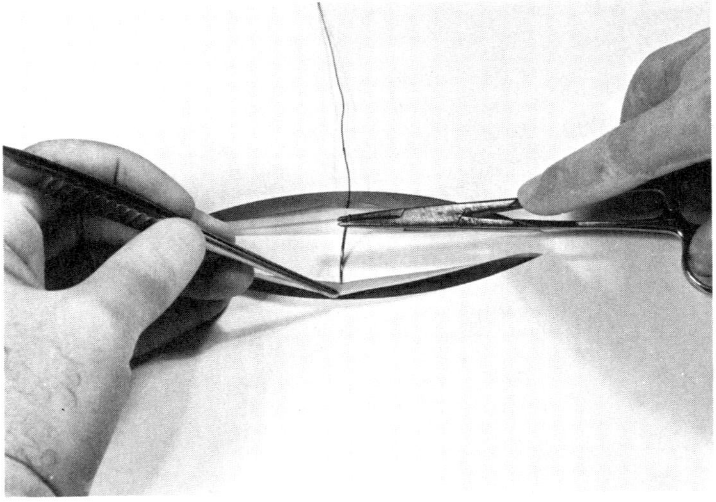

Figure 55. Step 3 use of forceps in suturing is lifting the near-side layer to be stitched to expose planned needle entrance site.

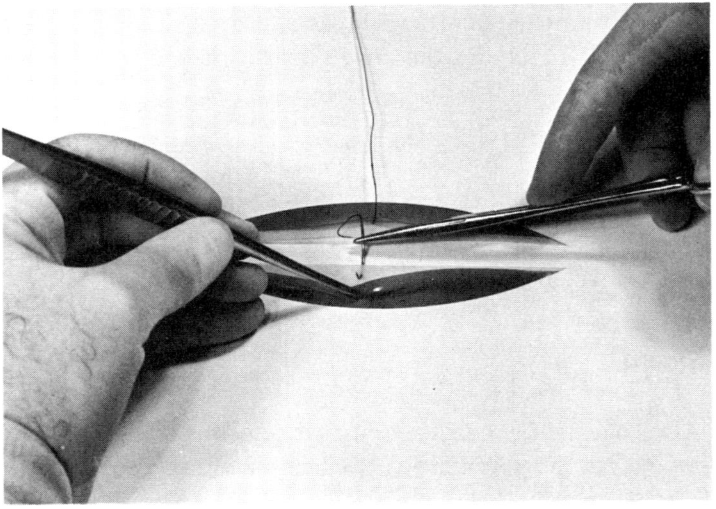

Figure 56. After needle entry on the near side, Step 4 is retracting the superficial layer with forceps to expose the needle exit site.

use of the forceps expands from mere stabilization of the layer being sutured, to an instrument of exposure, as well. The improved exposure makes for more accurate layer apposition, without inadvertent inclusion of a layer above or below that being sutured.

The expert use of tissue forceps makes the surgeon a two-handed operator.

Tissue forceps can be used in two ways during needle extraction. Forceps can be used to grasp the needle before releasing by the needle holder, or the forceps can hold the tissue on the needle during the needle holder release, to prevent distraction of the needle from the tissue. Use forceps with "teeth" to stabilize tissue more effectively on the needle; use "smooth" forceps to grasp needle more effectively for extraction.

If the tissue forceps are being used to extract a needle, apply the same principle of grasping the needle perpendicular to the shaft as when using a needle holder (Chapter 3). The perpendicular grasp is more secure than grasping with an oblique or parallel attitude. The perpendicular grasp also allows a mere rotation motion of the instrument to extract the needle, without changing the axis of the forceps.

In many situations, tissue forceps and clamps can be used interchangeably. A bleeding vessel may be either grasped by tissue forceps or clamped with a hemostat for cautery; a fascial plane may be grasped by either forceps or a clamp for traction to gain exposure. Forceps have an advantage over clamps as they can be more easily and quickly opened and closed, and the tension on tissue can be more precisely gauged than with clamps. Clamps, on the other hand, have the advantage of stronger grip and the ability to hold for an extended time without causing fatigue.

SUMMARY

Tissue forceps function as extensions of the thumb and opposing fingers. Hold the forceps between thumb and forefingers, with the shanks resting against the metacarpal-phalangeal joint of the index finger or in a pencil position.

When alternately using tissue forceps, as when sewing then tying, palm the tissue forceps while tying. In the palmed position hold the forceps with the sublimis muscles, not the profundus. Change the forceps from the "hold" to the "use" position with the palm down, allowing gravity to move the forceps away from the palm so the thumb and index fingers can easily regrasp the forceps in the proper position.

Approach the wound with the forceps from the side opposite the instrument in the other hand. This allows freer mobility of use. Maneuvers that require wrist flexion should be started in extension and vice versa, whereas maneuvers that require supination should be started in pronation, and vice versa.

Forceps are used to hold, retract, stabilize, extract, pack sponges, and pass ligatures. For maximum exposure and stability while suturing, move the tissue forceps from superficial to deep layers on the far side of the wound, then from deep to superficial layers on the near side.

Forceps can be used to secure tissue on the needle during extraction or to grasp the needle for extraction. Grasp needles perpendicular to the shaft for accurate extraction by rotating on the axis of the forceps.

Chapter 5

Knot Tying

In tying knots, one of the ends of the suture is frequently attached to a needle or ligature reel, so that there is a free end and a fixed end. During practice always put a clamp on one end of the ligature so as to become accustomed to taking the free segment in the proper hand. Otherwise, in the operating room you may grab the free end with the wrong hand, then need to pull the needle, holder, and surgeon through the knot.

It is impolite to pull the surgeon through the knot.

The common knot used in surgery is the square knot. The square knot consists of two mirror-image half hitches, one placed on the other; in contrast to a granny knot, which is made of two identical half hitches. A half hitch is one revolution of one end of a ligature around the other. The revolution is made in two half-revolutions. The first half is made by crossing the ligature segments; the second by putting the free end through the loop made by the crossing. The second half of the revolution is done differently by laymen and surgeons. Laymen poke the suture through the loop. Surgeons poke a finger or fingers through the loop, then grasp and bring the free end through. Control is thereby maintained by keeping hold of the free end during the manipulation. In proceeding through the following knot-tying maneuvers, stay aware that you are merely revolving the free segment a single turn around the fixed one.

Understanding what you are doing is better than just memorizing steps.

Square knots are tied by three methods: two-handed, one-handed, and instrument. Each method has advantages in specific applications.

The Two-Handed Square Knot
(Tied "Right-Handed")

Note that in the so-called "right-handed" tying, the manipulation is done with the left hand, which holds the fixed segment, and the right hand merely holds, lets go, and regrasps the ligature. Many right-handed surgeons tie left-handed, grasping the free end with the left hand. An advantage of left-handed tying, besides the manipulation being done with the dominant right hand, is that a surgeon tying his own knots during suturing does not need to change hands with the needle holder to do a two-handed tie. If you desire to learn to tie left-handed, look at the figures in a mirror and reverse the words "right" and "left" in the text.

Left-handed knot tying may, in reality, be right-handed.

The two-handed knot has the advantage of the greatest precision in maintaining constant tension on the suture during the tying process.

The Half Hitch

Step 1.   Grasping the Ligature   Grasp the uncrossed segments so that the ends are toward the little finger aspect of the hands (Fig. 57). Hold the free segment between the right index finger and right thumb. Hold the fixed segment by the middle, ring, and little fingers, so as to leave the left thumb and index finger free for subsequent manipulation (Fig. 57). Make the segments an optimal length for tying. The half hitch will be formed in the left hand, so the right will need to do its manipulation farther from the wound. Therefore, leave that portion of suture between the point to be tied and the hand, longer on the free than the fixed segment.

Don't shortchange yourself on the free end of a tie.

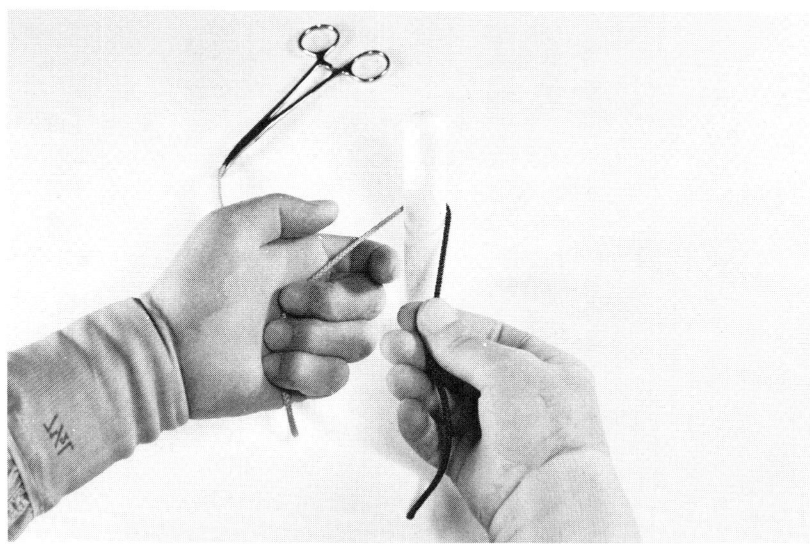

Figure 57.   Step 1 of the half hitch is grasping the uncrossed segments of the ligature. Follow text.

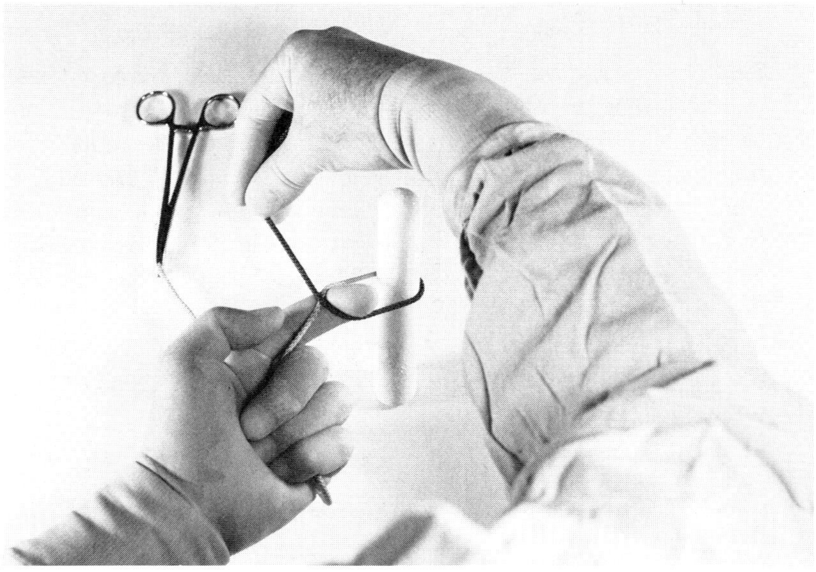

Figure 58. Step 2 of half hitch: crossing the ligature on the left index finger.

Step 2. Crossing the Ligature on the Left Index Finger Bring the free segment between the left index and middle fingers and wrap it one half turn around the index finger, thus making a cross on the left index finger (Fig. 58).

Step 3. Poking the Left Thumb Through the Loop Bring the very tips of the left thumb and index finger together (Fig. 59). Then push the thumb through the loop, replacing the index finger. The cross is now on the left thumb (Fig. 60).

Step 4. Bringing the Free End Through the Loop Place the free segment between the tips of the left thumb and index finger (Fig. 61) and rotate the free end through the loop (Fig. 62). Let go of the free end with the right hand.

Step 5. Tightening the Half Hitch Take hold of the free segment with the right hand and pull down the half hitch (Fig. 63).

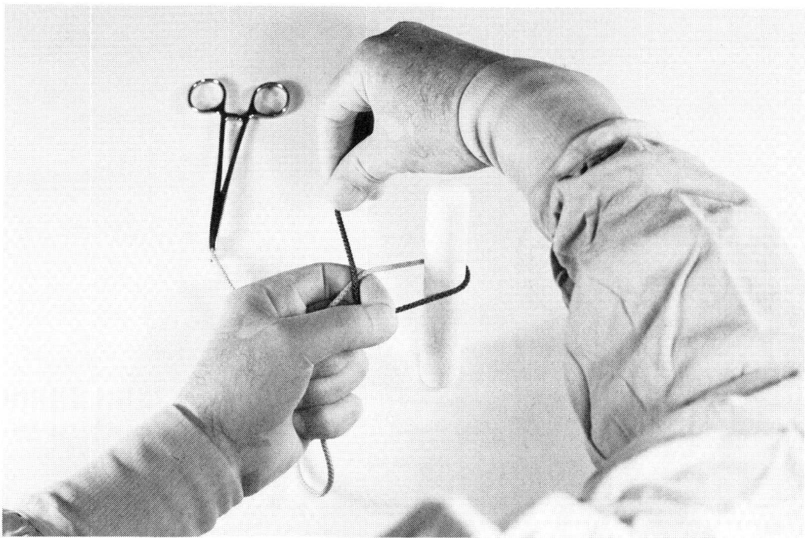

Figure 59. Begin Step 3 of half hitch by bringing tips of left thumb and index finger together within loop formed by cross.

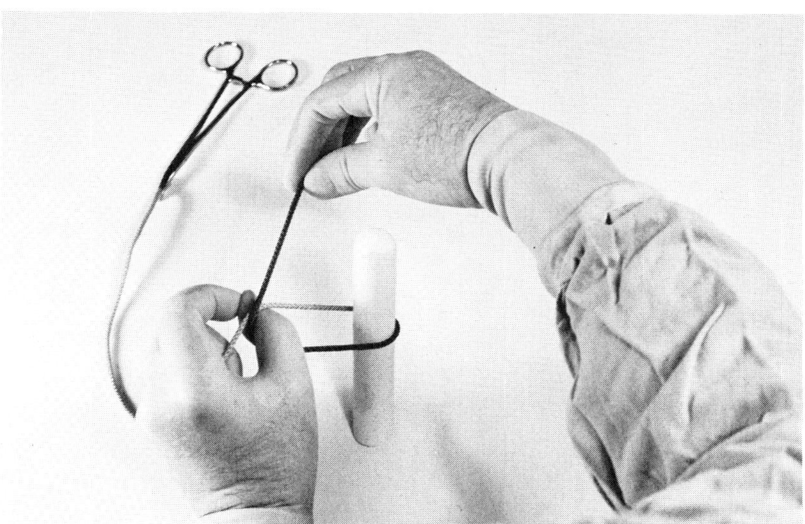

Figure 60. Complete Step 3 of half hitch, pushing thumb through the loop, transferring the cross onto the left thumb.

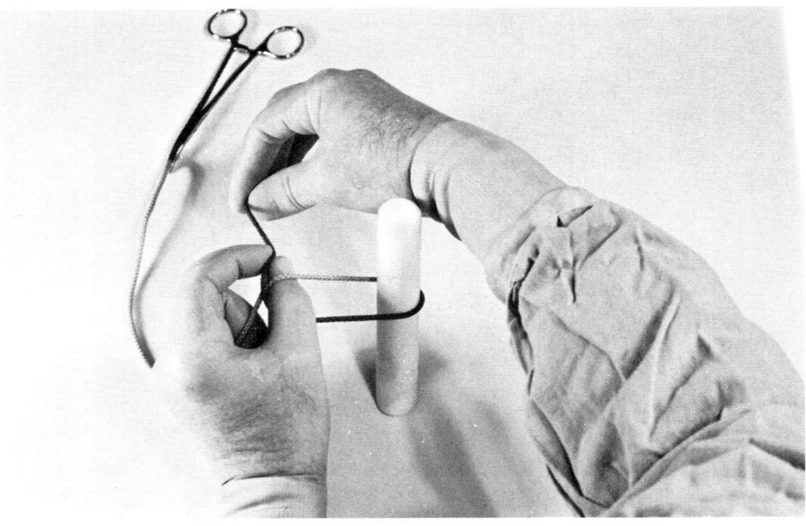

Figure 61. Begin Step 4 of half hitch by placing the free segment between left thumb and index finger.

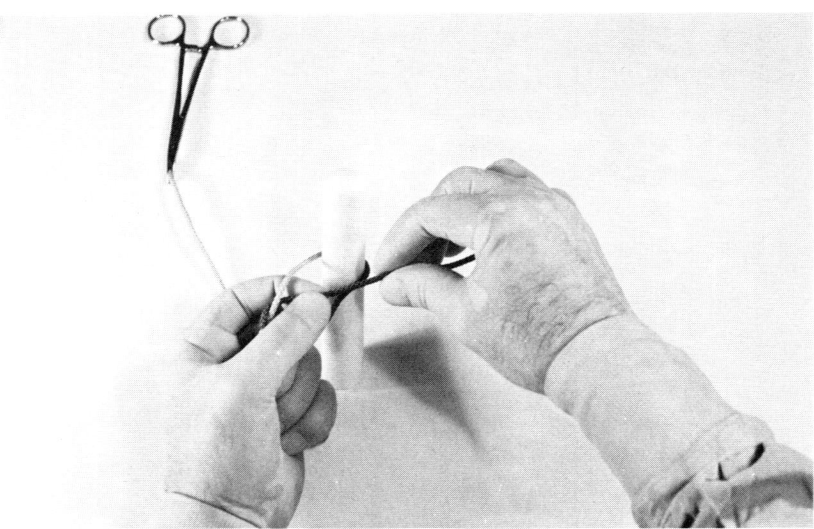

Figure 62. Complete Step 4 of half hitch by rotating free end through the loop and releasing free end with right hand.

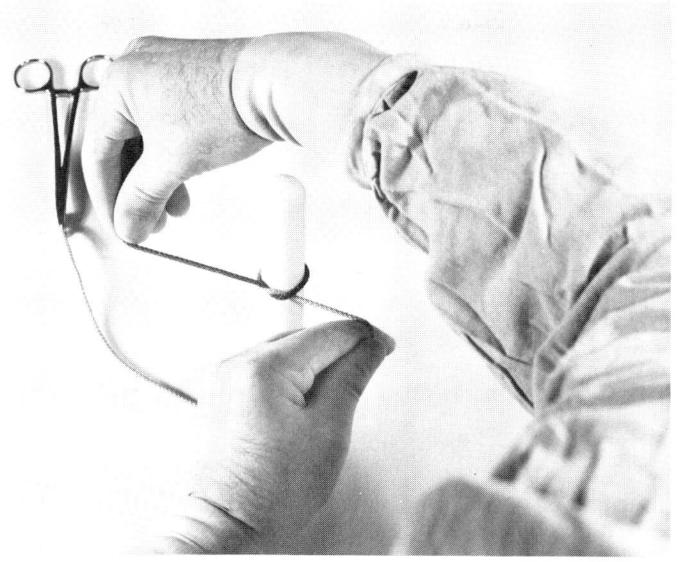

Figure 63. Step 5 tightens the half hitch. Follow text.

In wrapping one end of a ligature around the other to form a half hitch, the ends finish on opposite sides from where they started. To lay the tie flat, therefore, the segments must be crossed from their original position (Fig. 63). To assure that each segment makes a half turn around the other, exert equal tension on the two segments. Unequal tension would form a slipknot by causing one segment to form a complete revolution around the other straight one. Unequal tension may also stress the tissue being tied. It is important to pull the two segments so that they form a straight angle with one another, not an obtuse angle. A straight angle puts all of the tension in the knot. An obtuse angle puts a vector of unnecessary tension on tissue. When working in a deep wound it is necessary to carry one or the other segments into the wound over an index finger, in order to form the straight angle.

Cross the segments, not your hands.

The Mirror-Image Half Hitch

Step 1. Grasping the Ligature Continue holding the ligature, as when finishing the first half hitch, with the fixed segment on the palmar surface left index finger. Bring the tips of the left thumb and index finger together, than rotate the left hand so that the fixed segment enters the palm over the thumb (Fig. 64).

Step 2. Crossing the Ligature on the Left Thumb Bring the free segment between the left index finger and thumb and wrap it one half turn around the thumb, making a cross on the thumb (Fig. 65).

Step 3. Poking the Left Index Finger Through Loop Bring the tips of the left thumb and index finger together (Fig. 66). Then push the index finger through the loop, replacing the thumb. The cross is now on the index finger (Fig. 67).

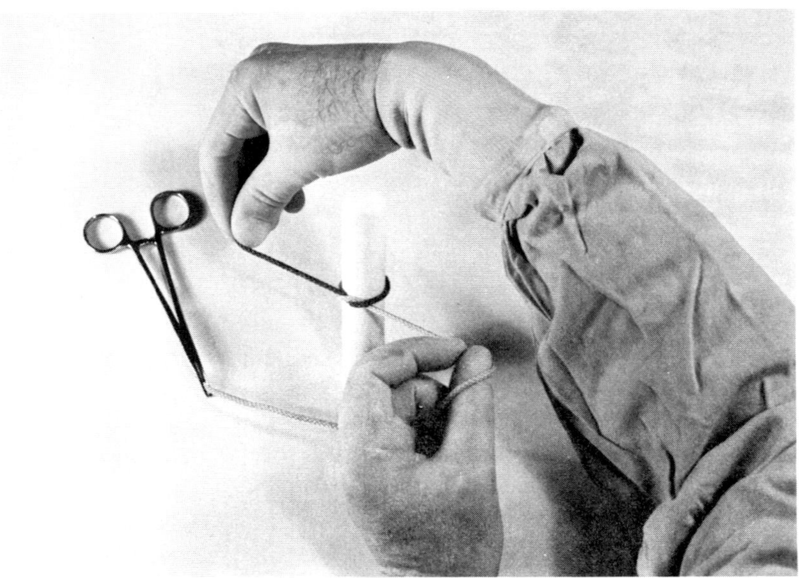

Figure 64. Step 1. To form the mirror-image half hitch continue grasping the ligature and bring the fixed segment over the left thumb and into the palm. Follow text.

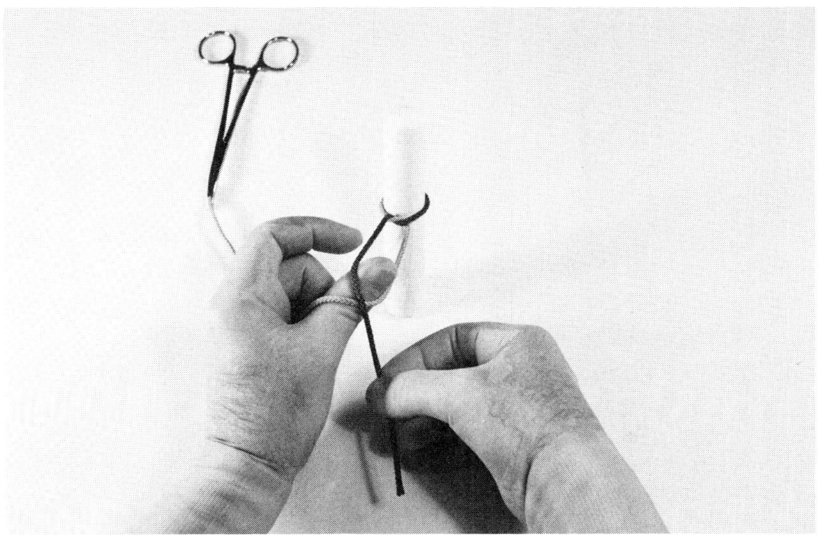

Figure 65. Step 2 of the mirror-image half hitch crosses the free segment over the left thumb.

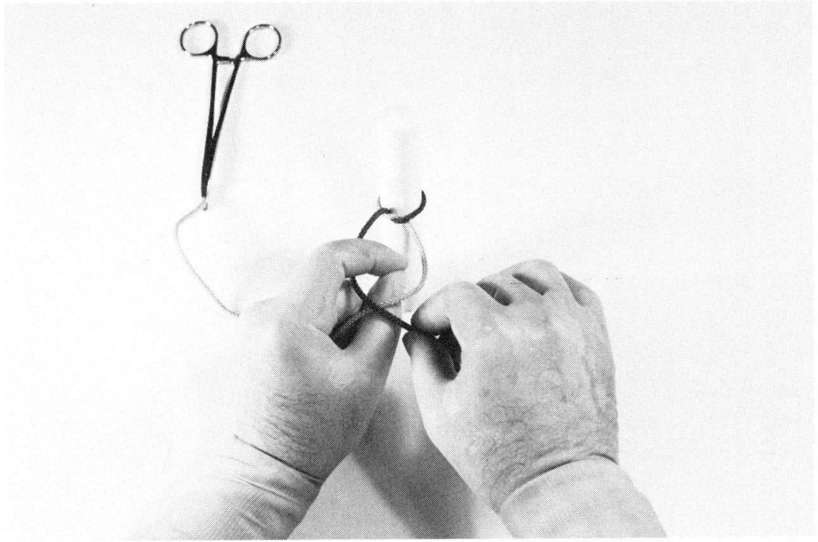

Figure 66. Begin Step 3 of the mirror-image half hitch by bringing left thumb and index finger together inside the loop.

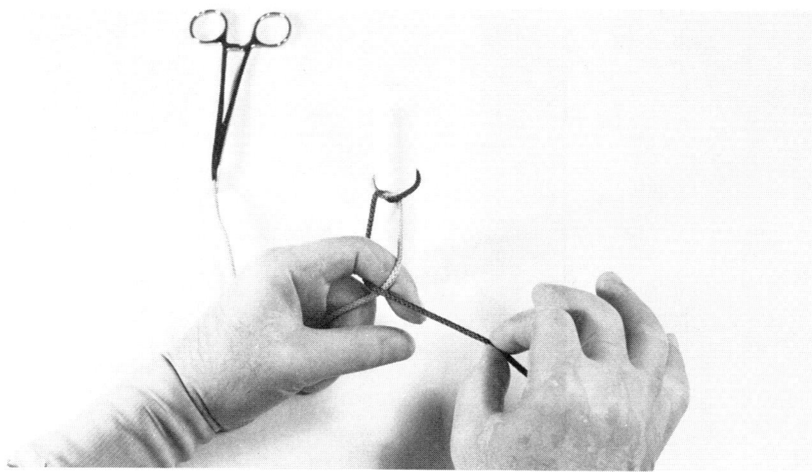

Figure 67. Complete Step 3 of the mirror-image half hitch by replacing the thumb with the index finger inside the loop.

Step 4. Bringing the Free End Through the Loop   Place the free segment between the tips of the left index finger and thumb (Fig. 68) and rotate the free end through the loop (Fig. 69).

Step 5. Tightening and Squaring the Knot   Take hold of the free end and establish tension with the right hand before the left hand releases. To square the knot, have the segments uncrossed from the starting position (Fig. 70).

The One-Handed Knot

The one-handed knot is so named because all of the maneuvering, including releasing and regrasping the free end, is done with one hand. The other hand merely holds the fixed segment taut. One-handed knots have the advantage of allowing more speed in tying, but have less tension control of the segments.

One-handed is really two-handed.

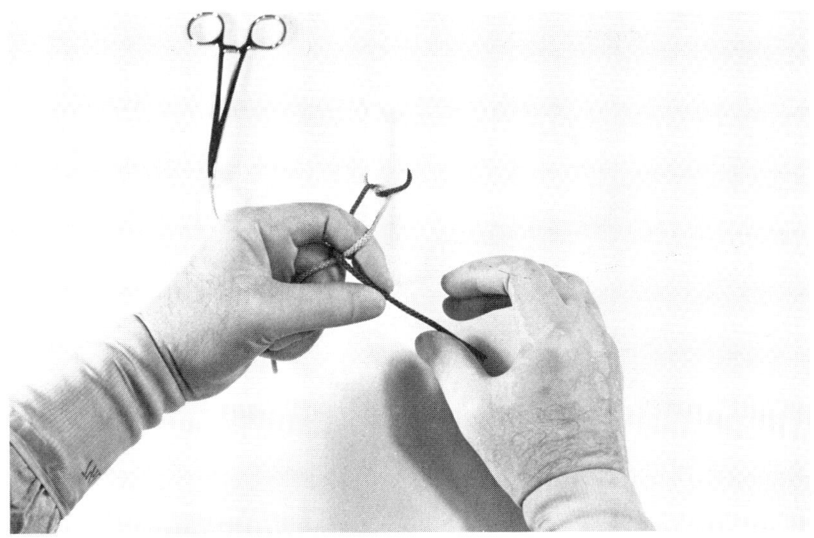

Figure 68. Begin Step 4 of the mirror-image half hitch by grasping the free segment between left index finger and thumb.

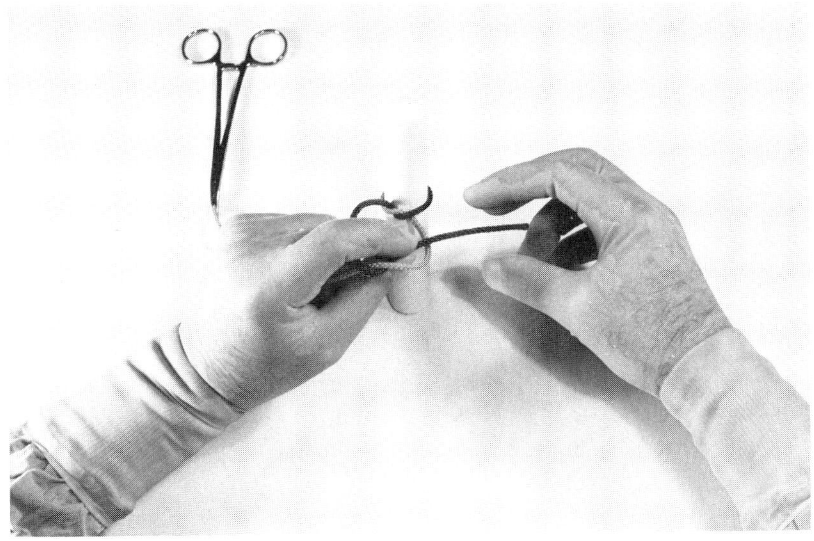

Figure 69. Complete Step 4 of the mirror-image half hitch by rotating the free end through the loop.

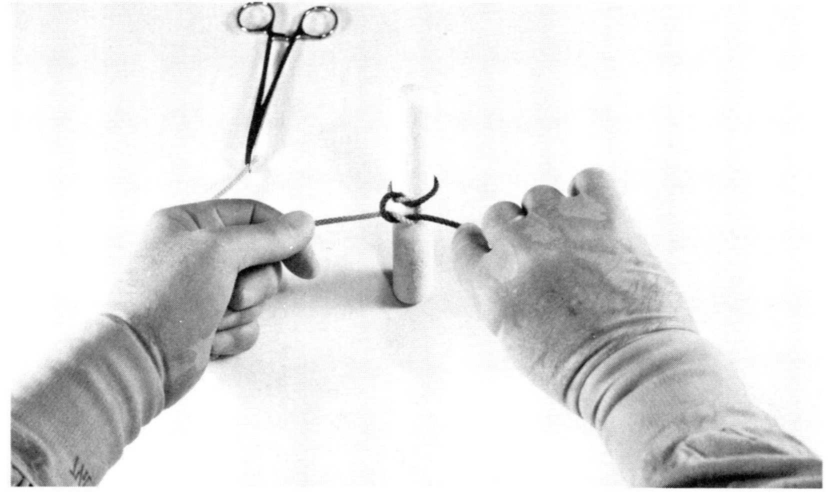

Figure 70. Complete the mirror-image half hitch with Step 5, tightening and squaring the knot with hands uncrossed.

The maneuvering is done with the left hand so that a surgeon tying his own knots during suturing can continue to hold the needle holder in his right hand. The one-handed knot is made by forming a loop around the left middle and ring fingers, putting the free end between these fingers, which then grasp the free end and bring it through the loop.

Step 1.

Grasp the free segment between the left thumb and index finger tips 3 in. from the end. Orient the end toward the palm (Fig. 71). Depress the thumb-index finger grasp of the ligature toward the little finger side of the palm.

Step 2.

Bring the fixed segment between the left ring and little fingers and wrap it one half turn around the middle and ring fingers (Fig. 72).

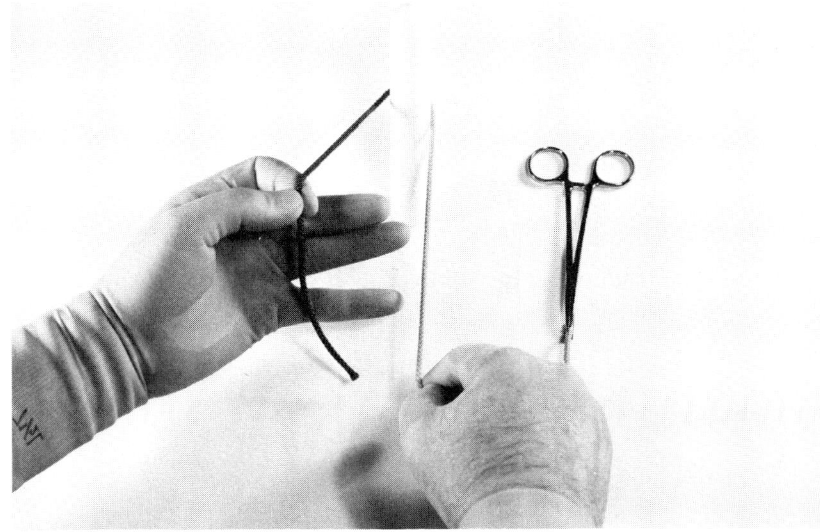

Figure 71. Step 1 of the one-handed knot is to grasp the free segment between left thumb and index finger three inches from the end.

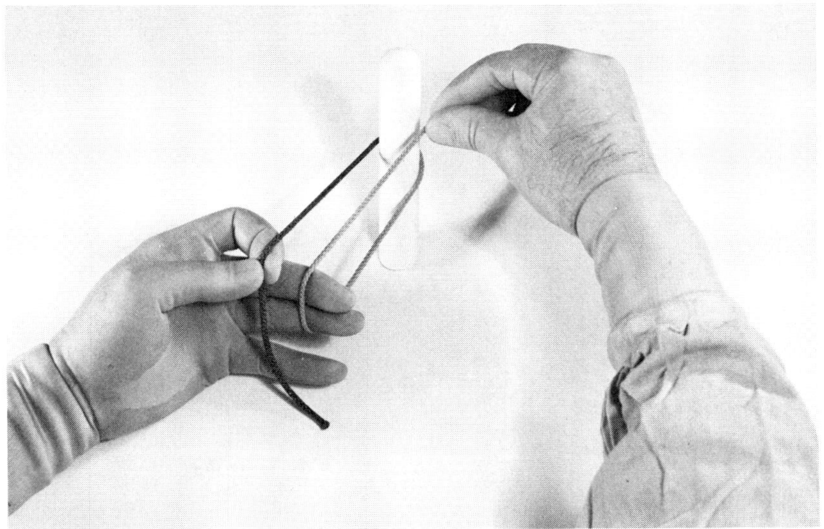

Figure 72. Step 2 of the one-handed knot wraps the fixed segment one half turn around the left ring finger and middle finger.

Step 3.

Flex the left ring finger (Fig. 73) so that the dangling free end can be grasped between the left middle and ring fingers (Fig. 73).

Step 4.

Let go of the left thumb-index finger grasp and pull the free end through the loop with the middle and ring fingers (Fig. 74).

Step 5.

Set the half hitch (Fig. 75) with hands crossed.
An alternate method of forming the first half hitch in one-handed knot tying is the "index finger," or "one-finger," half hitch.

Step 1. Alternate Method

Hold the free segment between the left thumb and middle finger with the segment entering the palm over the radial aspect of the index finger (Fig. 76).

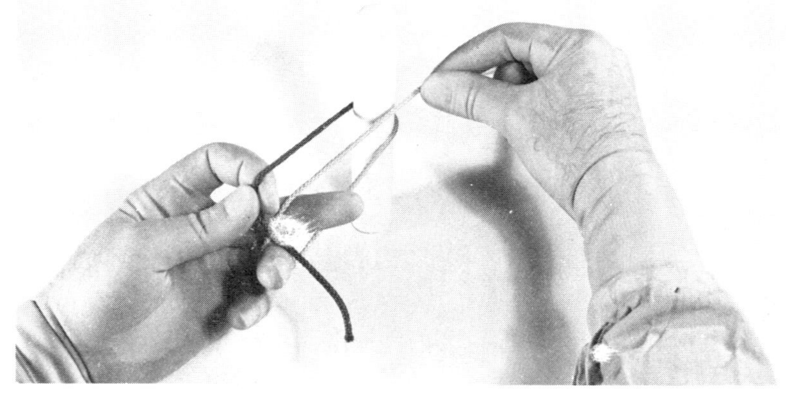

Figure 73.   Step 3 of the one-handed knot grasps the dangling free end between the left middle and ring fingers.

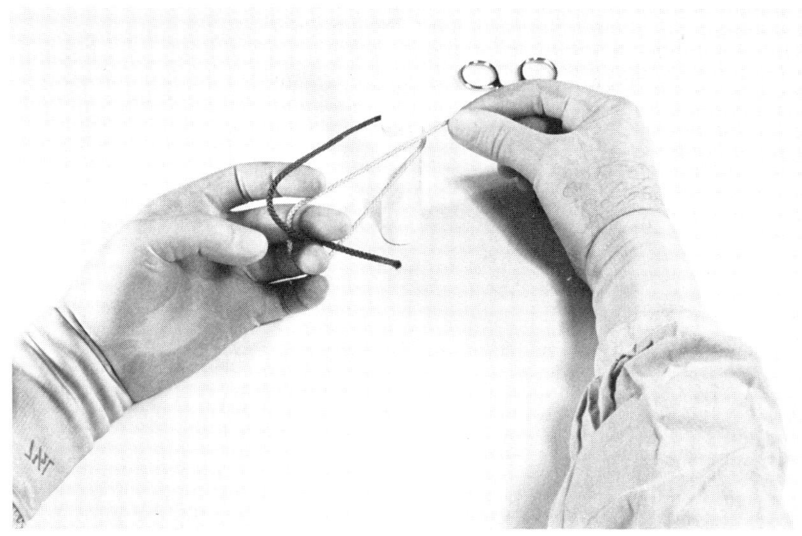

Figure 74. Step 4 of the one-handed knot pulls the free end through the loop with the left-hand middle and ring fingers.

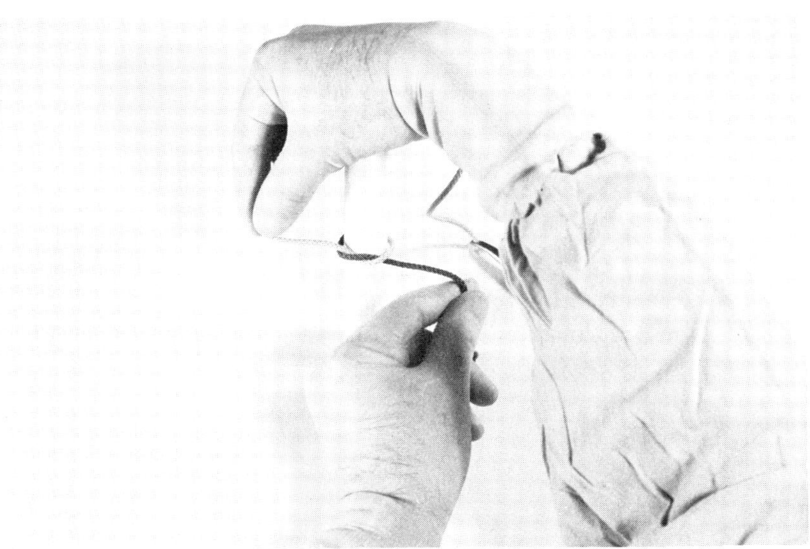

Figure 75. Step 5 of the one-handed knot sets the half hitch with hands crossed.

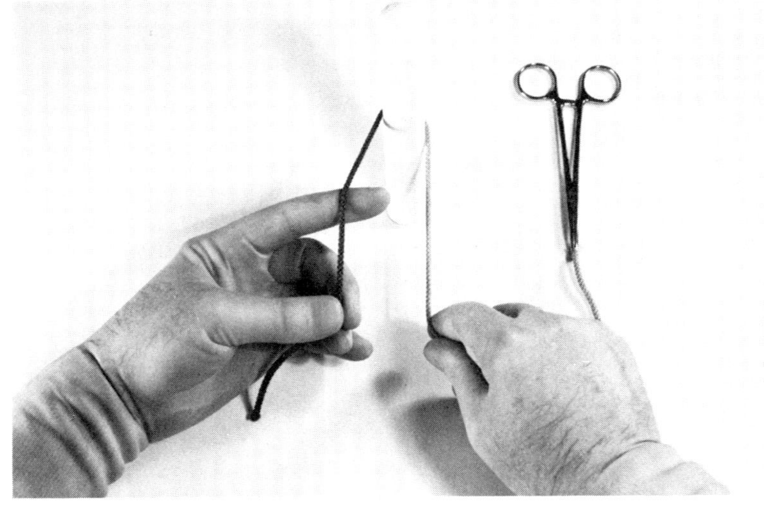

Figure 76. An alternate way to form first half hitch of one-handed knot, Step 1 is to pass free segment over index finger and grasp the material with left thumb and middle finger.

Step 2.

Bring the fixed segment between the index and middle fingers and wrap it one half turn around the index finger, making the loop around, and the cross on, the left index finger (Fig. 77).

Step 3.

Flex the left index finger to trap the fixed segment of the loop and pull 2 cm additional fixed length into the loop, thereby moving the cross 1 cm away from the index finger (Fig. 78).

Step 4.

Extend the left index finger in such a way as to trap the free segment between the cross and the thumb-middle finger grip. Pull the trapped segment through the loop (Fig. 79).

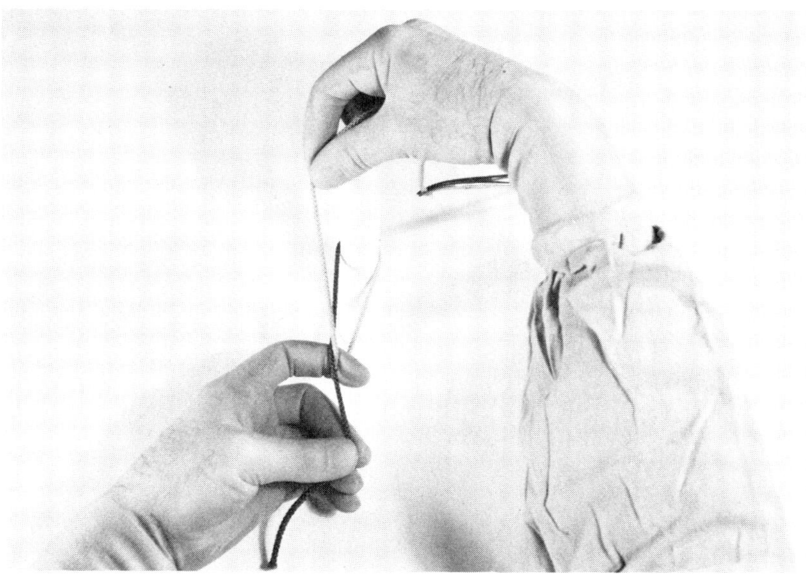

Figure 77. In alternate first half hitch of one-handed knot, Step 2 crosses fixed segment over index finger.

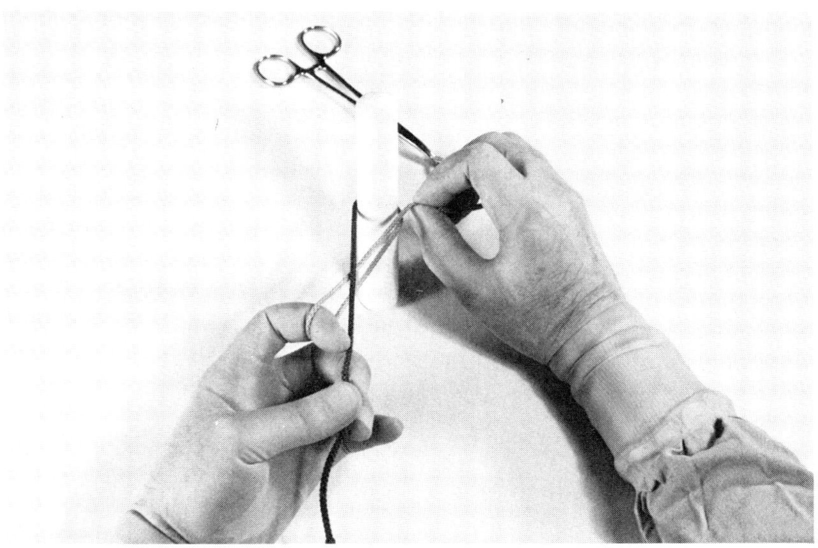

Figure 78. Step 3 of alternate first half hitch of one-handed knot; follow text.

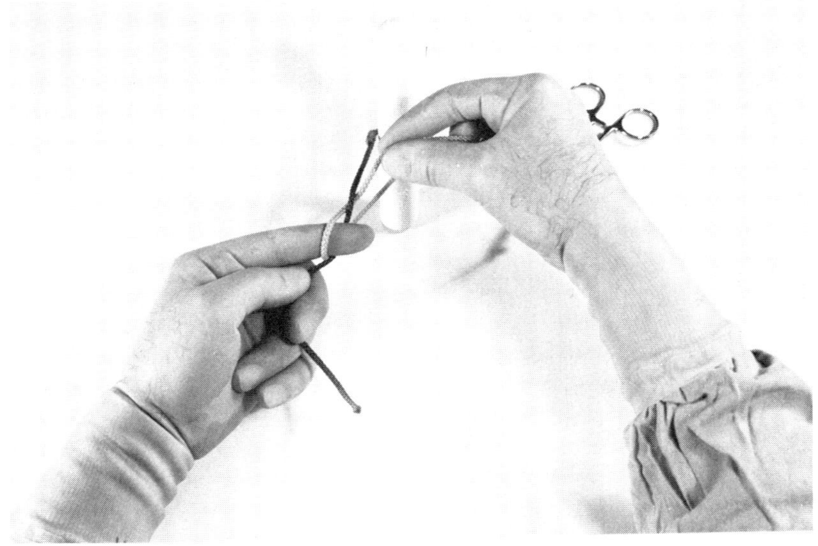

Figure 79. Step 4 of alternate first half hitch of one-handed knot: pull the trapped free segment through the loop.

Step 5.

Grasp the free segment between the left thumb and index finger as the thumb and middle finger release it (Fig. 80). Then set the half hitch with the segments crossed (Fig. 81).

The fact that this first half hitch of the one-handed knot has an alternate method is a clue that it is hard to do and is less controlled than the second mirror-image half hitch. In tying an interrupted suture, which has two free ends, there is advantage in using only the mirror-image one-handed half hitch, alternating between the left and right hands. The alternating hand method of throwing the easy second or mirror-image half hitch is conducive to the most rapid knot tying.

When there is more than one accepted method, there is usually no good method.

Flashy! Eh?

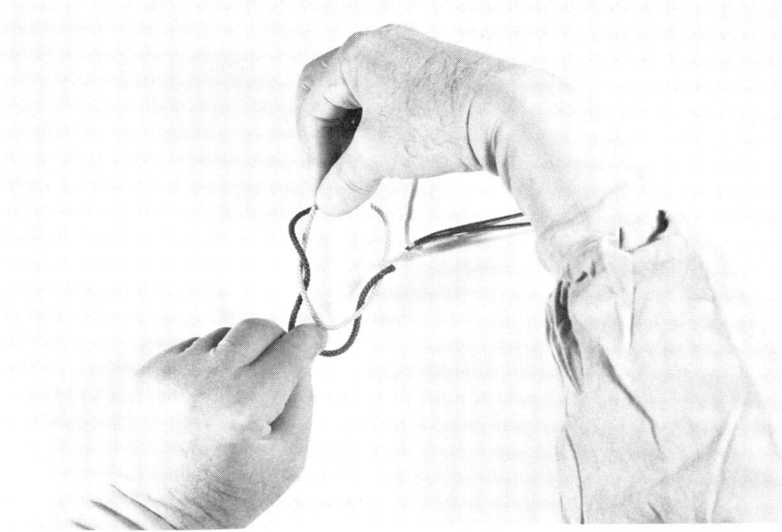

Figure 80. Begin Step 5 of alternate first half hitch of one-handed knot; follow text.

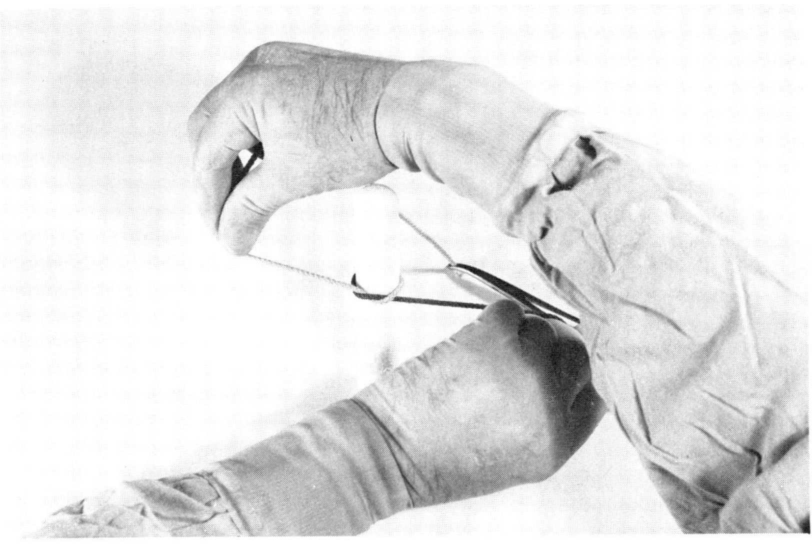

Figure 81. Complete Step 5 of alternate first half hitch of one-handed knot by setting half hitch with hands crossed.

The Mirror-Image One-Handed Tie

Step 1.

Grasp the free segment between the left thumb and index finger as it ends with the first one-handed half hitch (Fig. 75) or as it ends with the one-finger tie (Fig. 81). Make the free end in the palm between the left ring finger and the little finger (Fig. 82).

Step 2.

Bring the fixed segment between the index and middle fingers, and wrap it one half turn making a loop around the left middle and ring finger with a cross on the palmar surface of the ring finger (Fig. 83).

Step 3.

Flex the left middle finger and trap the free segment between the middle and ring fingers. Grasp the free end between these fingers (Fig. 84) and let go of the thumb-index finger grip (Fig. 85).

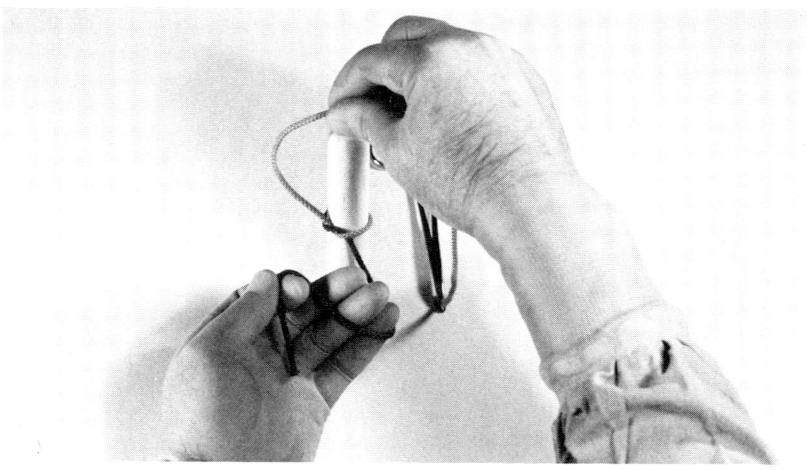

Figure 82. Step 1 of the mirror-image one-handed tie.

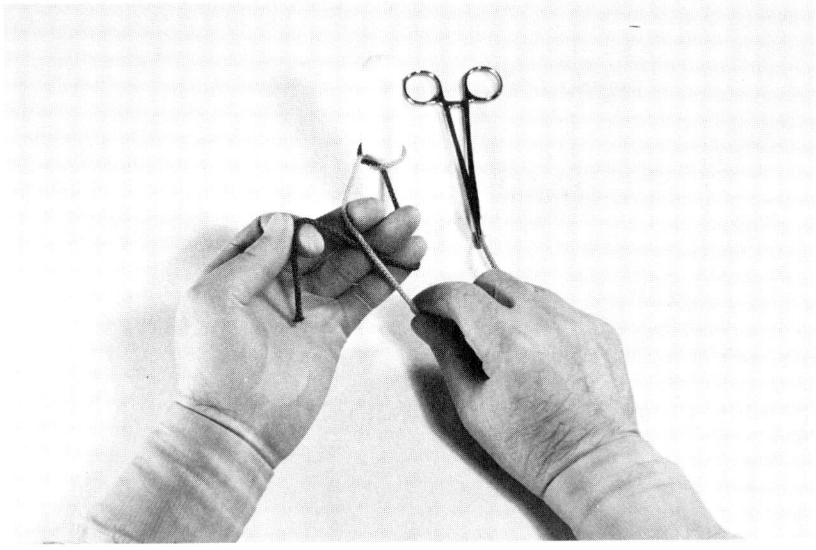

Figure 83. Step 2 of the mirror-image one-handed tie.

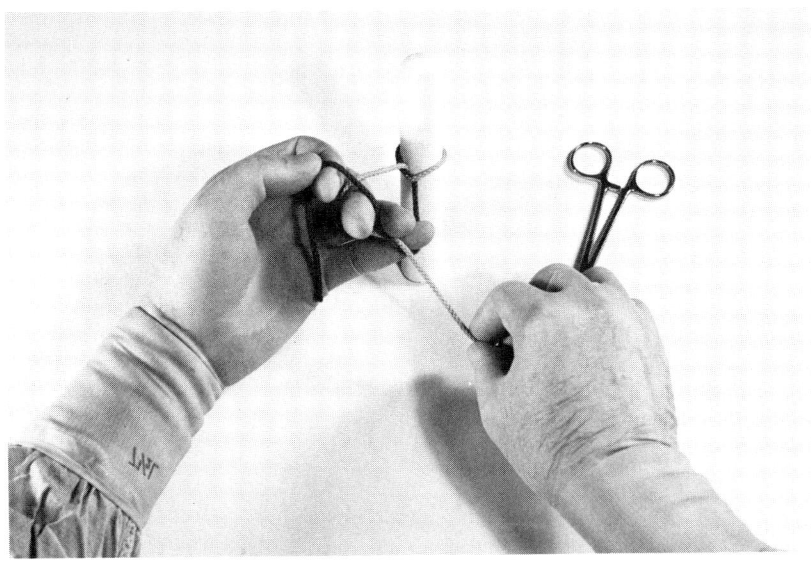

Figure 84. Begin Step 3 of the mirror-image one-handed tie by trapping the free segment between middle and ring fingers.

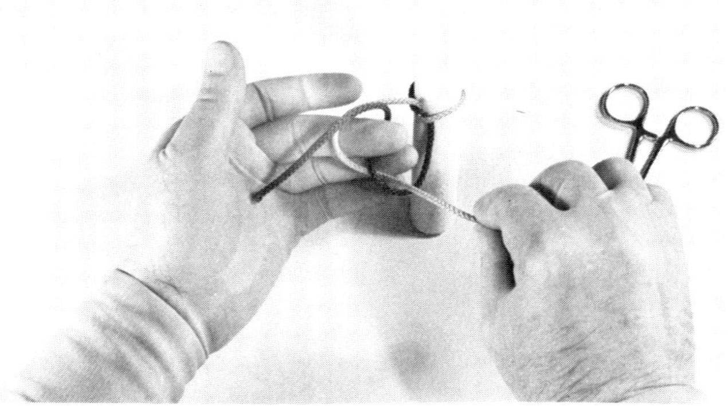

Figure 85.   Complete Step 3 of mirror-image one-handed tie by releasing free end from the thumb–index finger grip.

Step 4.

Pull the free end through the loop with the middle and ring fingers. Then set the half hitch (Fig. 86).

Instrument Ties

Instrument ties have the greatest advantage when the free segment to be tied is too short for the other methods.

Step 1.

Leave the free end ungrasped. Wrap the fixed segment clockwise one revolution around the jaws of a needle holder or clamp (Fig. 87).

Step 2.

Grasp the free end with the clamp and transfer the revolution to the free segment by pulling the free end through the loop with the instrument (Fig. 88).

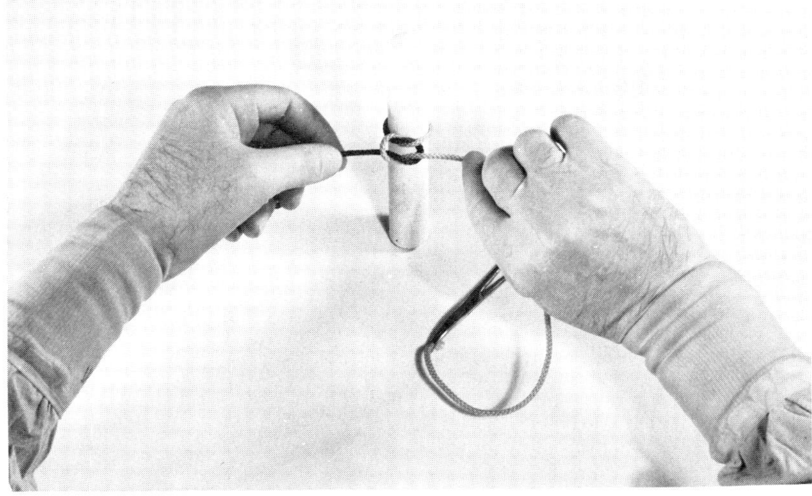

Figure 86. Step 4 pulls the free end through the loop and sets the mirror-image half hitch of the one-handed tie.

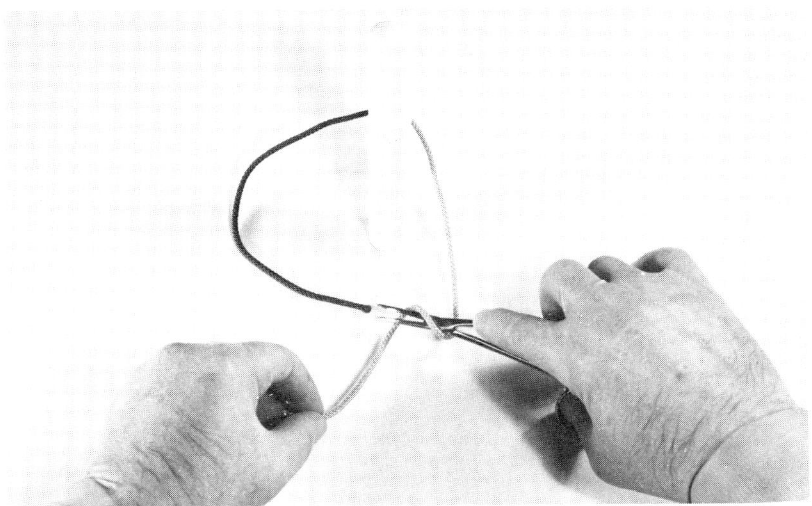

Figure 87. Step 1 of instrument tie leaves the free end ungrasped and wraps the fixed segment one revolution *clockwise* around the jaws of a needle holder or clamp.

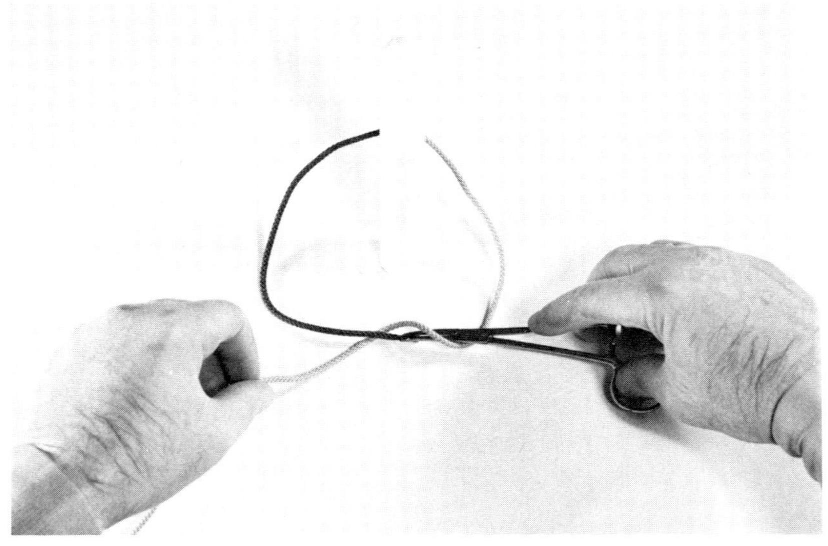

Figure 88.　In Step 2 of the instrument tie the clamp pulls the free end through the loop.

Step 3.

Set the half hitch with the segments uncrossed (Fig. 89). The mirror-image half hitch is formed the same way, except that the fixed segment is wrapped counterclockwise around the jaws of the instrument in the opposite direction from the first half hitch (Fig. 90). The knot is squared with segments crossed to the opposite sides (Fig. 91).

Slipknots

Knot tying requires special consideration when it is done under tissue tension. When tissue brought together by a half hitch is under tension there will be a tendency for the knot to loosen while the second half hitch is formed. Three methods of securing proper tissue apposition in such a case are: maintenance of continuous tension on both segments of the suture while tying the second half hitch, the tying of slipknots (nonsquared knots), and the use of a surgeon's knot.

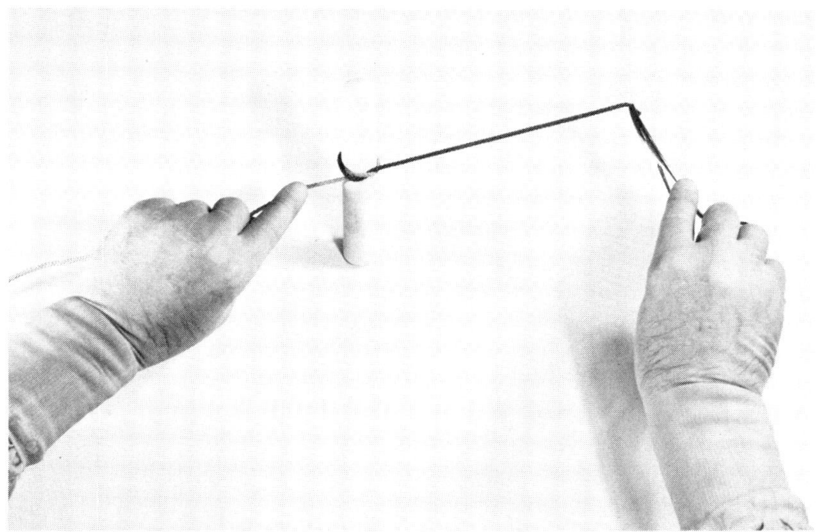

Figure 89. Step 3 begins by setting the half hitch with hands uncrossed.

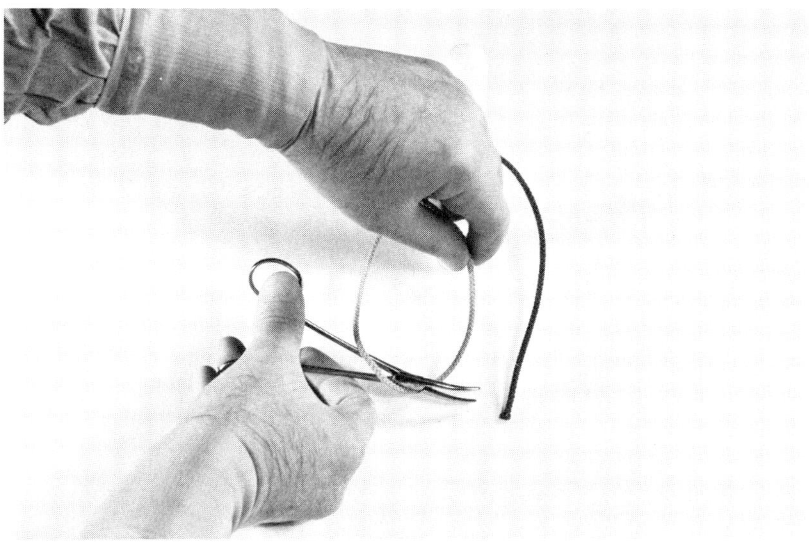

Figure 90. Step 3 of instrument tie continues by forming the mirror-image half hitch, in which the fixed segment is wrapped *counterclockwise* around the instrument.

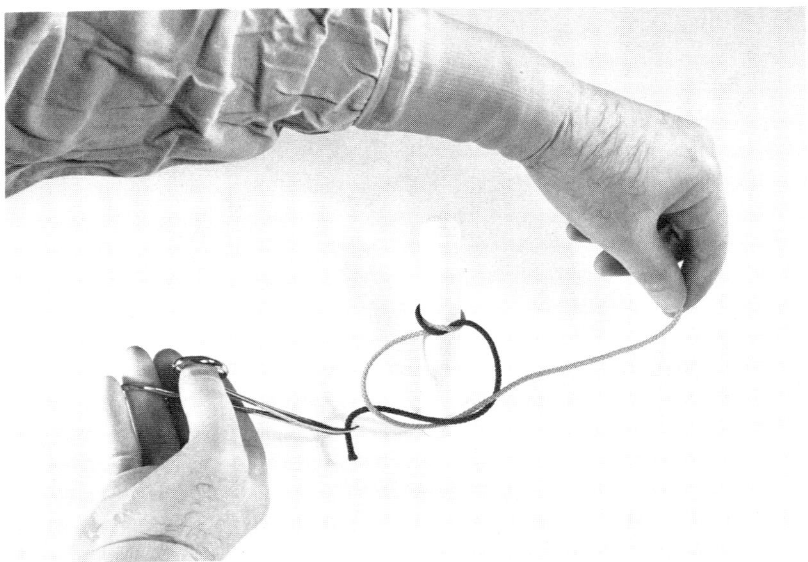

Figure 91. Complete Step 3 of instrument tie by squaring the knot with hands crossed.

Maintaining continuous tension on two segments of a ligature during the manipulation of the second half hitch takes practice and should be mastered. The most critical point, where tension is most likely to be lost, is between Steps 4 and 5 (Figs. 69 and 70). Tension must be established by the right hand before the left hand releases. Maintaining continuous tension is a useful method in many situations but has one mechanical disadvantage; the tension to prevent knot slippage is applied perpendicular to the distracting force of the wound. Such a perpendicular force vector added to the distracting force may, in some cases, be enough to tear tissue.

Learn from the mistakes of others; there won't be enough time to make them all yourself.

The slipknot method has a mechanical advantage in that only the force vector that tends to approximate tissue is applied to the knot. A slipknot is two half hitches, either mirror-image (square knot) or identical (granny knot), tied with greater tension on one segment than on the other. A square knot, contrary to popular opinion, slips almost as well as a granny does. A slipknot is made by not squaring the first half hitch (Fig. 92), then pulling on the fixed segment more than on the free segment after tying the second half hitch (Fig. 93). The greater tension on one segment keeps that segment straight; the half hitches remain as loops on that segment. The ability to slip depends on having one straight segment supporting both loops formed of the other segment. The slipknot is seated by pulling the straight segment with slightly more tension than the looped one, thus sliding the knot into position. Squaring is then done by reversing the strength of tension on the two segments. The slipknot can be very useful in restoring approximation of tissues when a square knot has been inadvertently tied too loosely. The knot, even though squared, can be turned into a slipknot by letting go of one end and tugging several times on the other to straighten out that segment. After getting the loops on the straight segment, the slipknot thus formed is slipped into place by pulling on the straight segment with greater tension than on the looped one. By such a method, most of the time a well-squared knot can be turned back into a slipknot, and vice versa.

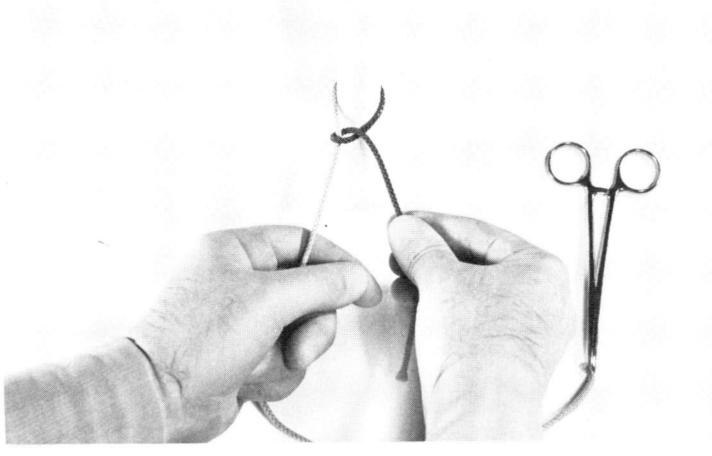

Figure 92.   In a slipknot, the first half hitch is not squared.

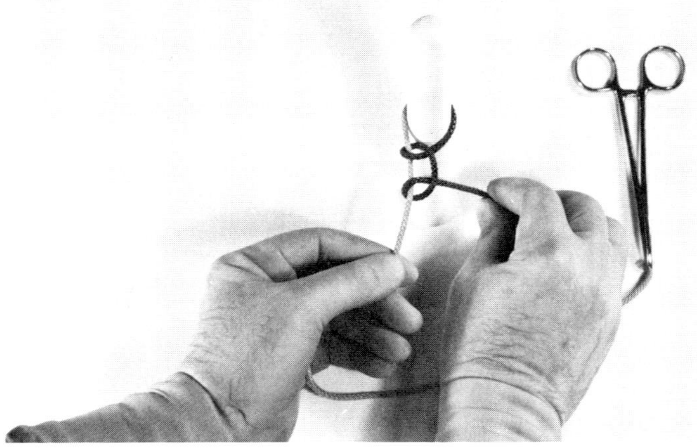

Figure 93. The second half hitch of a slipknot should be tied with greater tension on one segment than on the other. The half hitches remain as loops on the straight, tighter segment.

Most knots can be made to slip by letting go of one segment, then pulling on the other.

A surgeon's knot is merely one with a double half hitch for the first throw (Fig. 94), which can be locked by reversing the direction of pull on the segments (Fig. 95). After locking a surgeon's knot, the lock will stay if no tension is exerted on each segment. The double half hitch will not lock unless there is tissue beneath it to hold it. Tension on either segment will unlock the double half hitch. The second half hitch, therefore, must be tied with both segments loose to take advantage of the lock. Any tug during the placement of the second half hitch will unlock the double half hitch and allow tissue to separate.

The surgeon's knot is also useful for tying Christmas packages, as an assistant does not have to put his finger on the first half hitch.

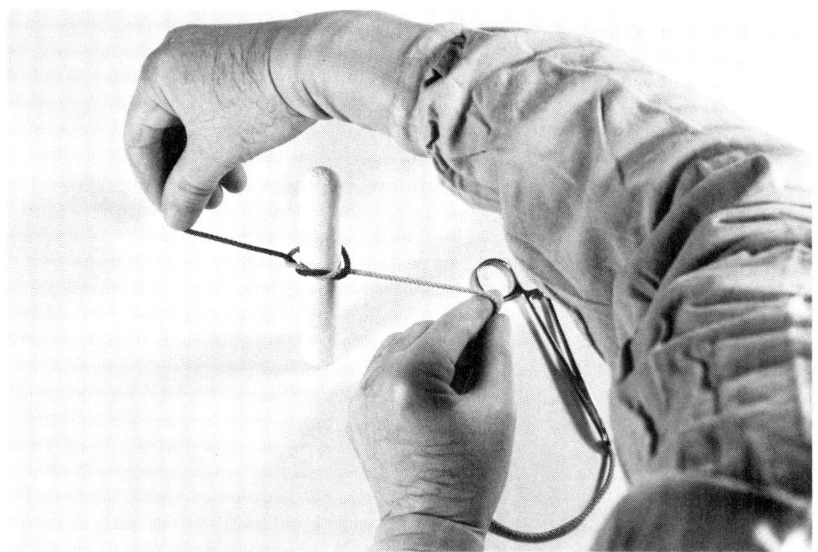

Figure 94. A surgeon's knot starts as a double half hitch.

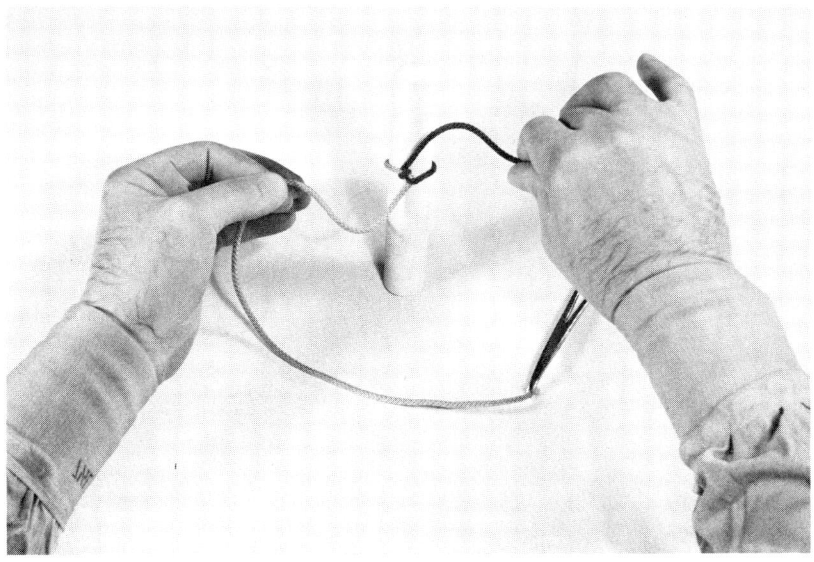

Figure 95. The surgeon's knot can be locked by reversing the direction of pull on the segments.

When tying knots, a short time spent maintaining tension after the first half hitch will allow tissue fluid to escape from beneath the tie and add security to the knot. In surgery usually a third half hitch, or throw, is placed for added security against the knot's later becoming untied. Generally, three throws are used on small bleeders and on ligatures in tissue which is not under tension. Four throws are used on large vessels and in tissue approximated under tension. Five throws are used on the heart, diaphragm, and other moving structures. Smooth, slippery suture material requires more throws for security than rough material such as cotton or silk. Knots squared well are more secure than those left as slipknots.

Fine and braided wire can be tied in the same way as other sutures. Heavy wires, on the other hand, need to be twisted rather than tied, as a tie would be so bulky as to be unacceptable. A secure twist is insured by making certain that each end winds equally around the other. Otherwise, one end left straight can easily be pulled out of the twists of the other. The weakest point and therefore the usual site of wire breaks is at the junction of the twist and the loop of wire in the tissue. Trying to pull tissue together by twisting the wire applies poor mechanical advantage to the tissue and maximal stress to the wire. Therefore, to prevent breakage, first pull up on the crossed ends to approximate the tissue, then twist to remove the slack from the wire. Three complete revolutions are adequate to secure a wire stitch. When using wire, thought should be given to bending and burying each wire

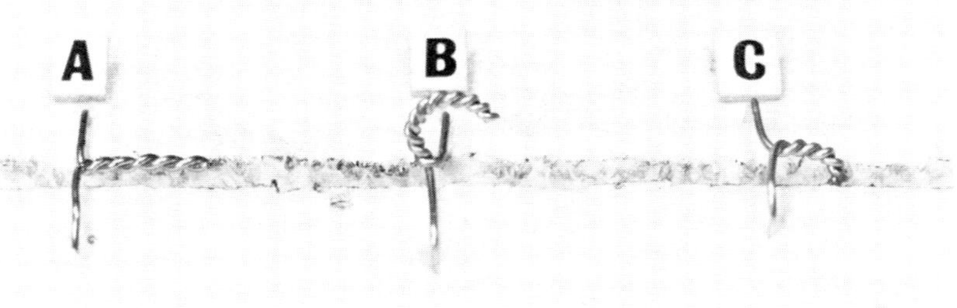

Figure 96. (A) If change in position occurs in buried straight wire ends, there is risk of exposure or too deep penetration of a free end. (B) For burying wire knots, curve the ends into two-thirds of a circle. (C) Turn the arc produced as in "B" down into the tissue or between bone edges.

knot or twist in such a way that it does not jeopardize any deep structure, and in such a way as to be unnoticeable to the patient after the wound is healed.

A sure method of burying wire knots is to first curve the ends into two-thirds of a circle (Fig. 96b), then turn the arc thus produced down into the tissue or between bone edges (Fig. 96c). If the knot then changes position, up to one-half a rotation, the free end cannot present more superficially or go deeper near vital structures, as may occur with straight wire ends (Fig. 96a).

Stapling devices, cautery, and more sophisticated innovations of the future will probably never completely eliminate the need for skill in the art of knot tying.

Chapter 6

Surgical Clamps

Surgical clamps have a great variety of uses, including hemostasis by the clamping of blood vessels; dissecting; retracting; tissue holding; ligature passing; suture tagging; and occluding of tubular structures, such as bowel or ducts, to prevent leakage of their contents. Some of these clamping techniques warrant special attention.

CURVED HEMOSTAT APPLICATION

Bleeding vessels can be secured with either of two clamping techniques: tip or jaw. The primary objective of the tip technique, shown in Figure 97, is to clamp the open vessel while including the minimum of surrounding tissue. Note that the tip is pointed toward the vessel. The vessel can then be ligated or cauterized, leaving a minimum of devitalized tissue within the wound.

The objective of the jaw technique, as shown in Figure 98, is to clamp the open vessel in the greater curvature of the jaw, with the tip pointing away from the vessel. Jaw clamping leaves the tip exposed beyond the tissue to trap the ligature more easily as it is passed around the vessel, thus facilitating placement of the ligature during tying.

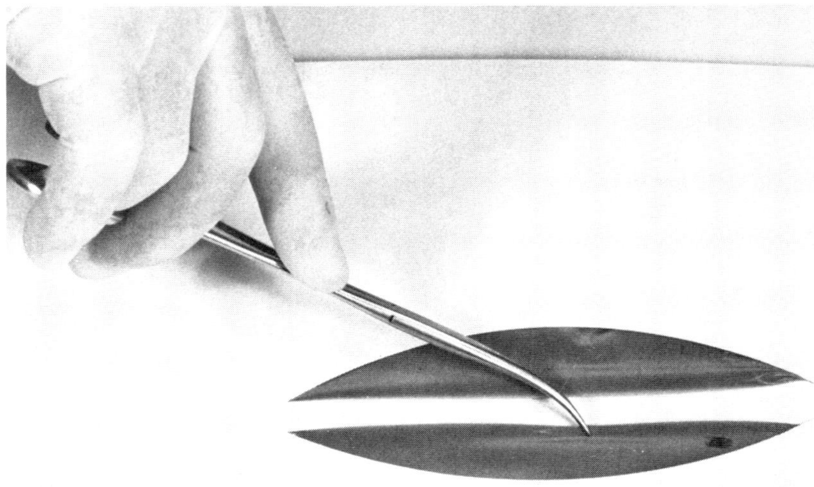

Figure 97. With tip of clamp pointing toward the open vessel, a curved hemostat is applied, using the tip technique to include a minimum of surrounding tissue.

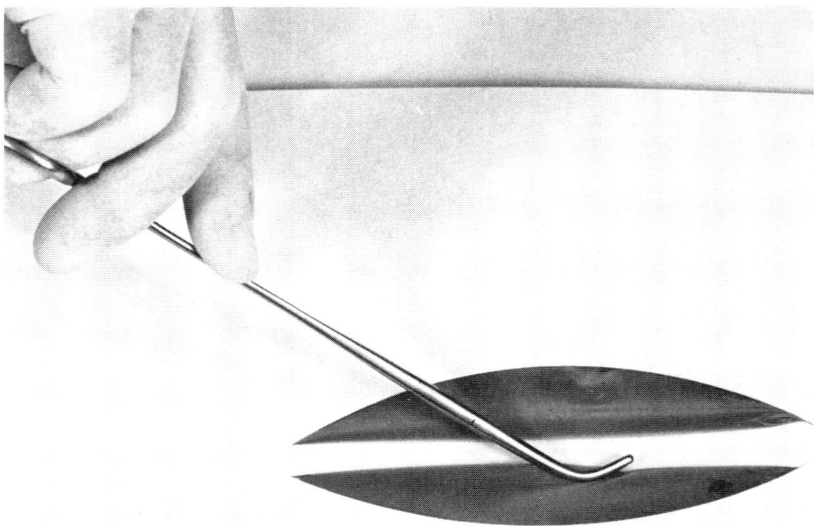

Figure 98. Jaw clamping, with the tip pointing away from the vessel, facilitates tying by trapping the ligature but devitalizes more tissue.

On a cut surface, clamping with the jaws includes more tissue than when clamping with the tip, thus sacrificing viable tissue for ease of knot tying. The tip method, which minimizes devitalized tissue in the wound, requires more coordination between the clamp operator and the ligator to trap the ligature. This is a minor inconvenience well worth the advantage of minimizing tissue devitalization.

Don't destroy tissue to save time. Speed should be a by-product of good surgical technique rather than a primary goal.

Clamping across uncut tissue planes for hemostasis before transection includes the same amount of tissue whether the clamp tips are pointed toward or away from the proposed cut (Fig. 99). Applying the clamp jaws with the tips pointed toward the intended cut and away from the vessel makes knot tying easier with no disadvantage (Fig. 100). The jaw technique is therefore superior when transecting vascular pedicles, omentum, mesentery, or other structures between clamps.

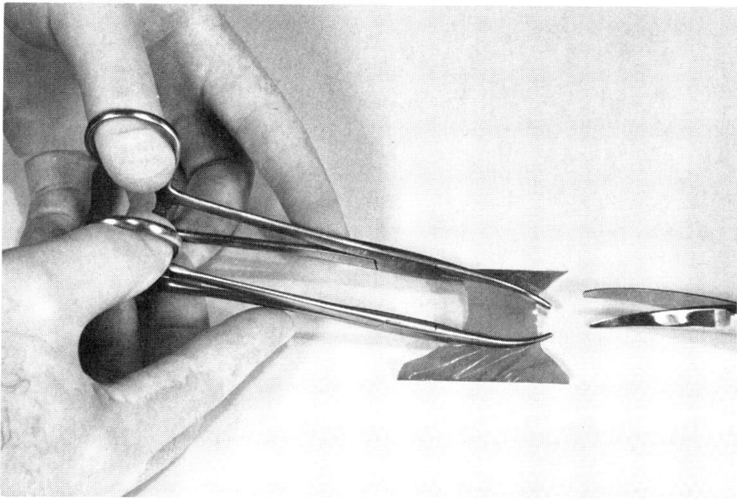

Figure 99. In clamping across uncut tissue pedicles, the same amount of tissue is included, regardless of the direction of the clamp tips.

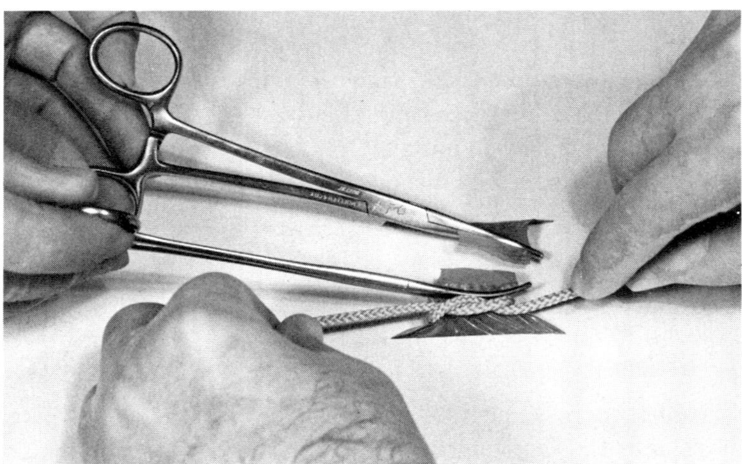

Figure 100. With clamp tips pointing toward the intended cut, tying is easier, with no penalty.

For greatest accuracy and security in applying hemostats, grasp a single instrument in your dominant hand with the thumb and ring finger in the finger rings, and the index finger on the shafts. In noncritical situations, where it's desirable to apply many hemostats or clamps in succession, you can save time by carrying several clamps in one hand (Fig. 101). Carry four to six hemostats on your ring finger; apply them one at a time by placing the thumb in the ring of the most superficial clamp, while continuing to palm the rest.

Palming several tools frees the instrument nurse from having to pass each separately. Carrying several clamps in one hand becomes a mere affectation and an impediment to accuracy when timesaving and decreased blood loss are not by-products. Palming is useful with other clamps, such as towel clips and tissue-holding clamps, where convenience and speed do not compromise accuracy.

MANIPULATION OF THE HEMOSTAT DURING VESSEL LIGATION

1. Hold the hemostat for encirclement by the ligature, as shown in Figure 102, without placing your fingers in the finger rings. This

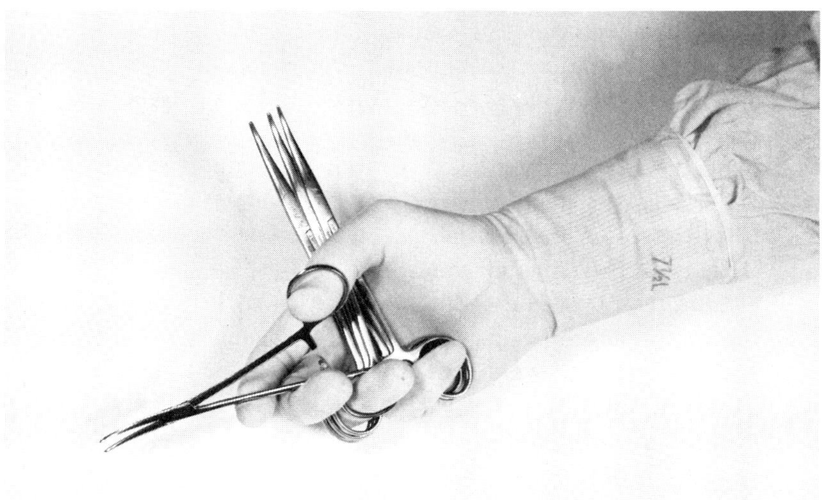

Figure 101. To apply many hemostats in succession, carry several clamps on your ring finger; apply one at a time by placing the thumb in the ring of the most available clamp.

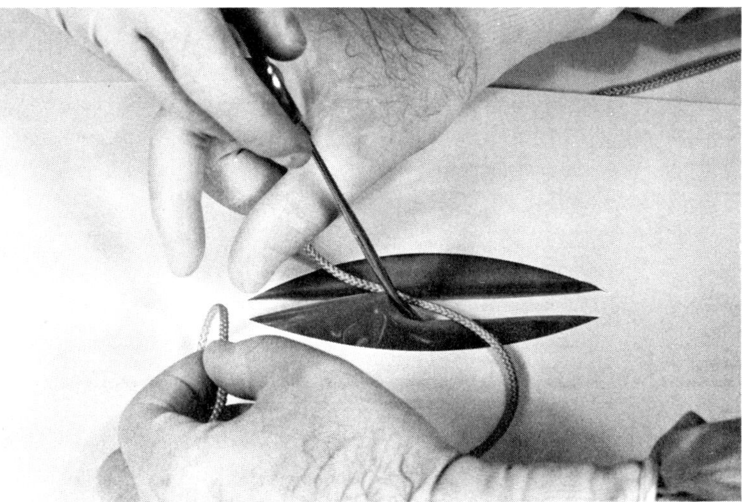

Figure 102. In Step 1 of vessel ligation, to allow optimal rotation for placing the tie, hold hemostat handles away from the wound, without fingers in the finger rings.

allows axial rotation to eliminate twisting of tissue and provides optimal rotation for placing the tie. The handles should be held away from the wound to avoid impeding the encircling hands of the knot tier.

2. Slide the surrounding ligature from the clamp to the tissue by depressing the handles away from the tier, and elevate the tip toward the tier as soon as the ligature has encircled the clamp (Fig. 103). The elevated clamp tip provides the knot tier with two alternatives: tying off of the tip or trapping the ligature beneath the clamp before tying.

3. If the knot tier ties off of the tip (Fig. 104), continue holding the hemostat as in Step 2 with the tip elevated. The knot tier can then place the half hitch he is forming beneath the tip and tighten it with a single maneuver. Tying off of the tip has one less step than when the ligature is trapped, and works best in superficial layers where both hands of the knot tier have access to the wound.

3. (Alternate Method). For added security in deep wounds or with critical ties, the tier can place the ligature around the tip of the

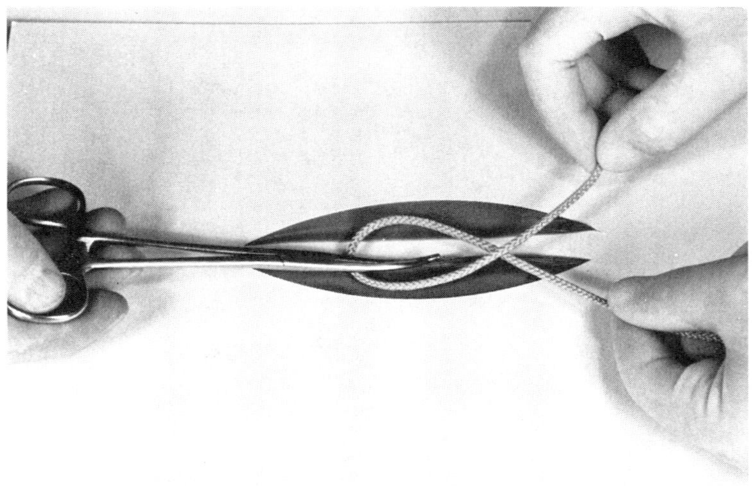

Figure 103. In Step 2 of vessel ligation, depress the handles away from the tier and elevate the tip toward the tier as soon as the ligature has encircled the clamp.

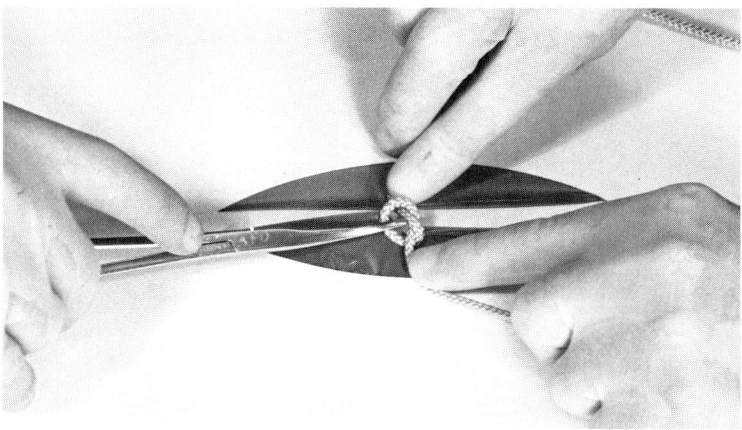

Figure 104. For Step 3 of ligation, with hemostat tips elevated, the half hitch can be formed beneath the tip and tightened wtih a single maneuver.

hemostat before tying. The one holding the clamp traps the ligature beneath the tip by gently pressing the clamp deeper into the wound and rotating the tip away from the tier. This maneuver will position the clamp to allow the knot to be tied on the side of the jaws, as shown in Figure 105. Failure to push the clamp tip

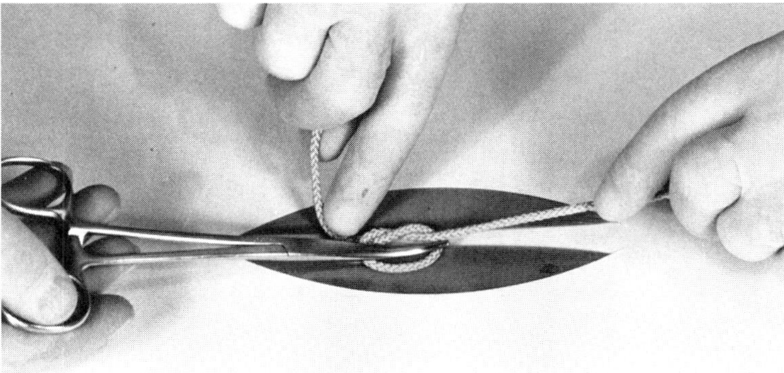

Figure 105. For an alternative Step 3, in deep wounds, the clamp tip is lowered and rotated away from the tier, to trap the ligature, so the knot can be tied on the side of the jaws.

away from the knot tier will cause the ligature to slip from beneath the tip, forcing the tier to tie off of the tip.

"Trap my ligature," not "Show me the tip," should be the plea of the operator who desires to pass the ligature around the tip before forming the knot.

Clamp Removal

While the operator tightens the first half hitch, gradually remove the clamp rather than snapping it off the wound. Gradual release of the clamp prevents the tissue from escaping while the first half hitch is tightened. The more secure and accurate grip to accomplish controlled release of a clamp in critical situations is the three-point grasp, with the thumb and index finger in the finger rings.

In noncritical situations, the thumb and ring finger grip has the disadvantage of limiting axial rotation to a proper attitude for knot tying by limiting forearm rotation. When more motion is needed than allowed by pronation and supination of the hand and forearm, the grasp has to be readjusted.

With the thumb and ring finger in the finger rings, you will also find it more difficult to discard a clamp than when the clamp rests free in the palm of the hand. The problem of release can be minimized by resting the clamp tip on a firm surface while the index finger exerts pressure on the closed shanks, pushing the clamp from the hand (Fig. 106). When removing hemostats in noncritical situations, palming the clamp, as shown in Figures 107 and 108, allows greater range and mobility to obtain optimal tip position in relation to the tissue and tier. Palming also allows effortless discarding of clamp, once it is removed.

To remove hemostats without putting fingers through the finger rings, whether using the right or left hand, it is the finger ring on the left which is grasped by the thumb. For right-handed removal, with the right hand in a neutral position, pinch the left ring between the thumb and ring finger (Fig. 107); disengage the lock by pressure of the

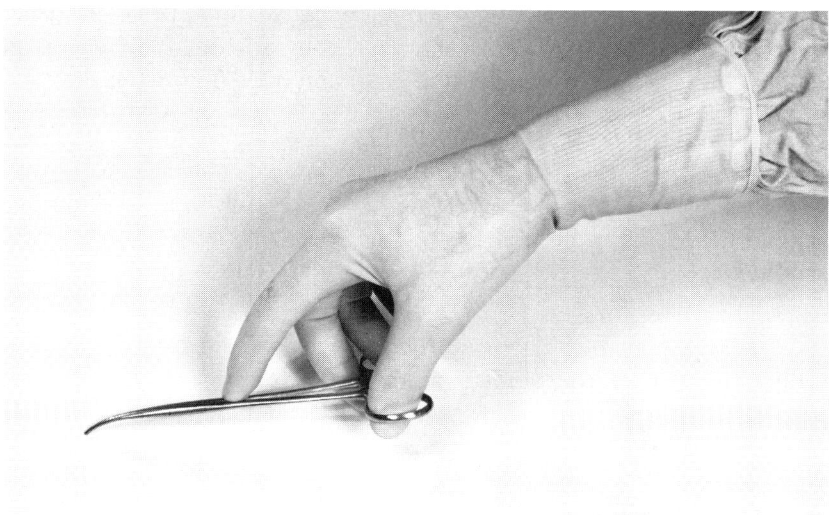

Figure 106. To aid discarding of clamp, rest the clamp tip on firm surface and push clamp from hand by pressing index finger on closed shanks.

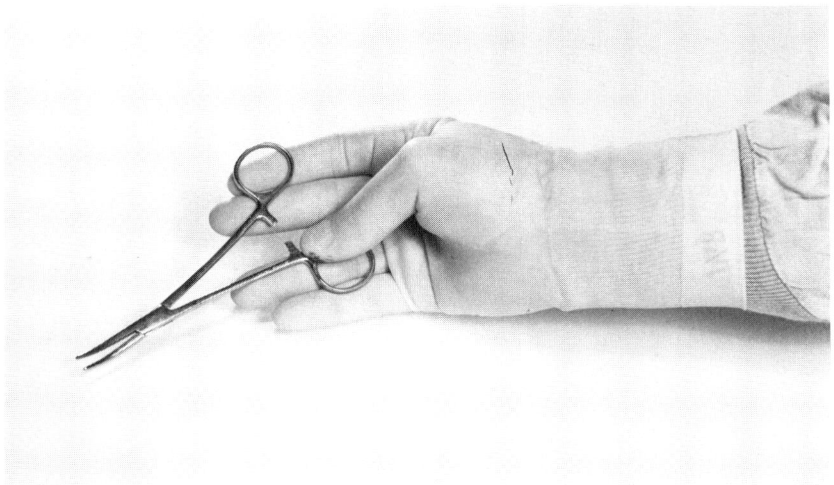

Figure 107. For right-handed removal of hemostat, with right hand in neutral position, pinch the left ring between thumb and ring finger; disengage the lock by pressure of the index finger on the right finger ring.

index finger on the right finger ring. For left-handed removal, grasp the left ring between the thumb and index finger (Fig. 108); disengage the lock by pressure of the middle, ring, and little fingers on the right finger ring.

Left-handed hemostat removal is most secure when fingers are not placed through the hemostat rings.

After removal of a hemostat, click it closed before setting it down or handing it back to the instrument nurse, to prevent entanglement with other instruments or sutures.

Steps in Tying Vessel Clamped by Hemostats

Because there are distinct advantages in tying "left-handed" as listed in Chapter 5, the follow description applies to "left-handed" knots.

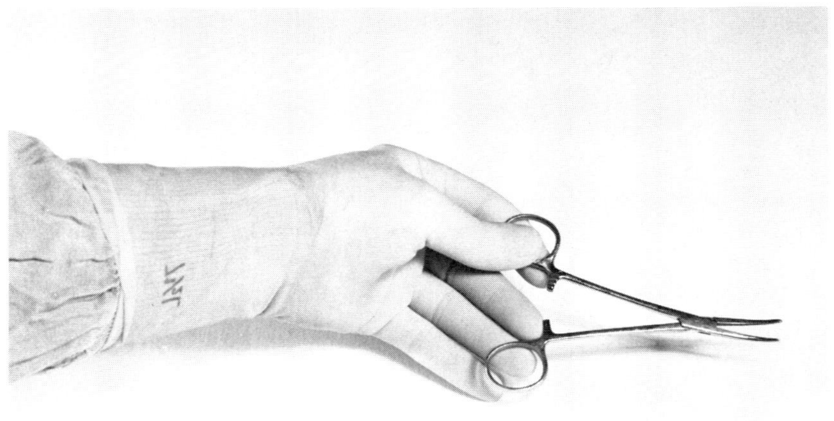

Figure 108. For left-handed removal of hemostat, grasp the left ring between the thumb and index finger; disengage the lock by pressure of the middle, ring, and little fingers on the right finger ring.

Step 1.

Pass the free end of the tie around the clamp. There are two options to this maneuver: One results in the suture being uncrossed, whereas the other results in the suture being crossed at the end of the pass.

In the uncrossed tie, the free end is passed counterclockwise behind the clamp by the right hand and received by the left hand, as shown in Figures 109 and 110. The only advantage of this technique lies in the slight time saved by a procedure with one less step.

In the crossed tie, the free end is grasped by the left hand and passed clockwise (Fig. 111) behind the clamp, received by the right thumb and index finger (Fig. 111), then transferred above the fixed segment back to the left hand (Fig. 112), resulting in a crossed ligature (Figs. 112 and 113). The crossed technique allows the first half hitch to be placed flat with the hands uncrossed in full view of the assistant during clamp removal (Figs. 114 and 115). This method also has the segments of suture uncrossed after the third half hitch, leaving the knot in full view of the assistant ready to cut the excess suture from the tie.

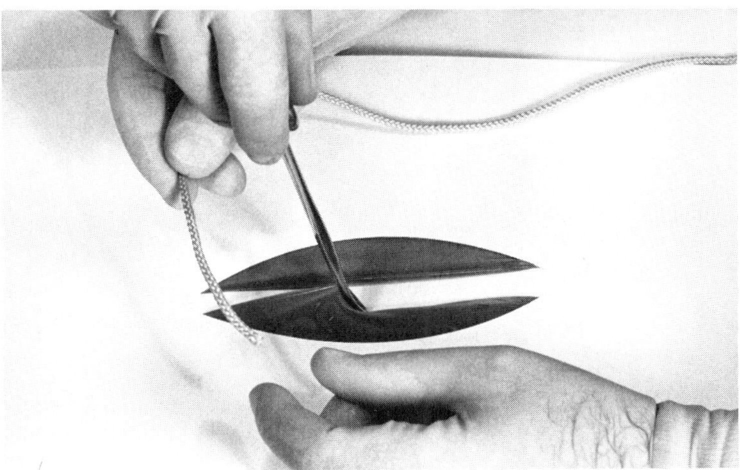

Figure 109. To begin the uncrossed tie of a vessel clamped by hemostats, the free end of the suture is passed by the right hand counterclockwise behind the clamp.

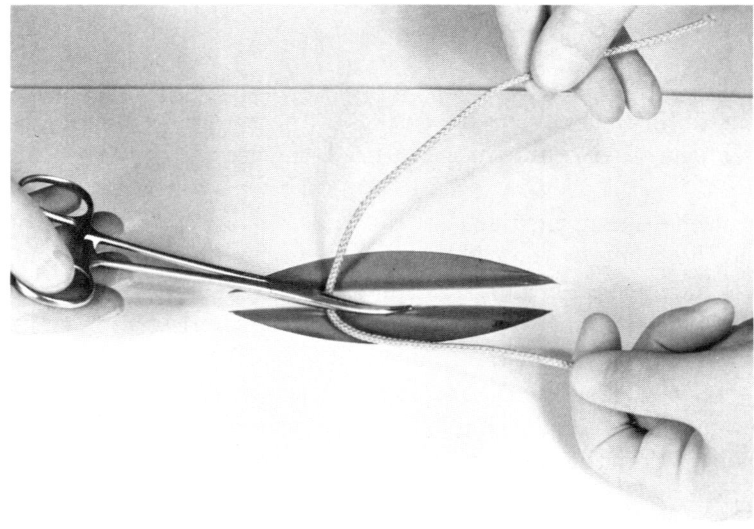

Figure 110. Continuing the maneuver started in Figure 109, the left hand receives the suture and pulls it behind the clamp.

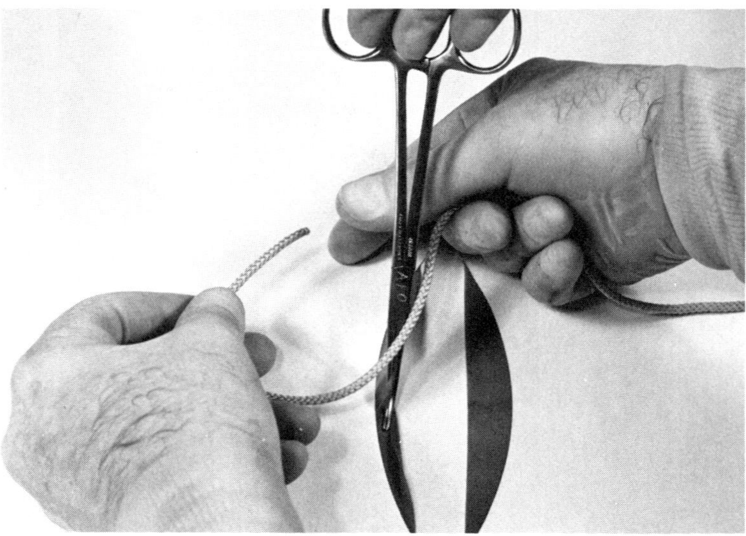

Figure 111. In the crossed tie, the free end is grasped by the left hand and passed clockwise behind the clamp, to be received by the right thumb and index finger.

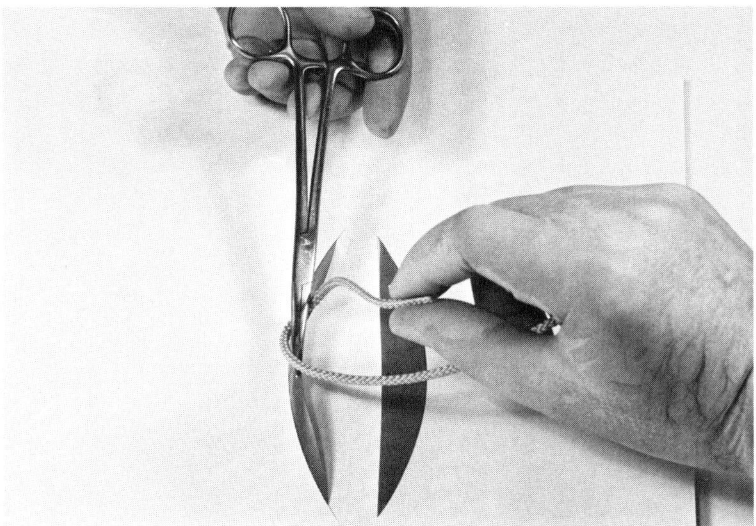

Figure 112. Continuing the maneuver started in Figure 111, the free end grasped by right thumb and index finger is to be drawn leftward above the fixed segment.

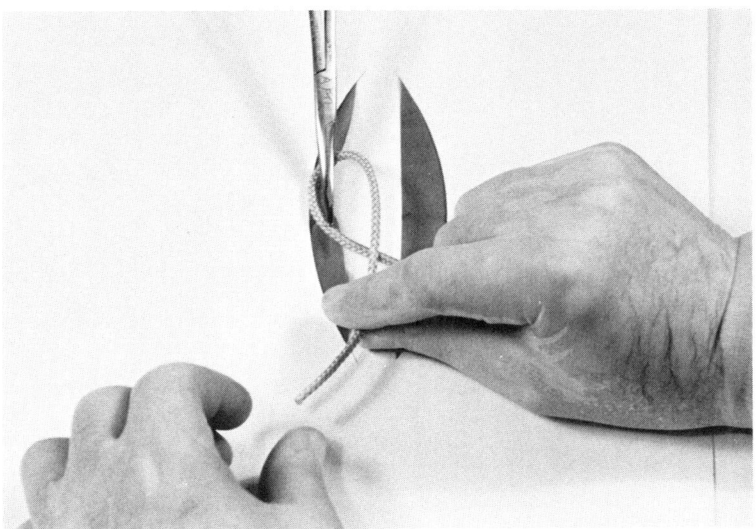

Figure 113. The left hand grasps the crossed ligature.

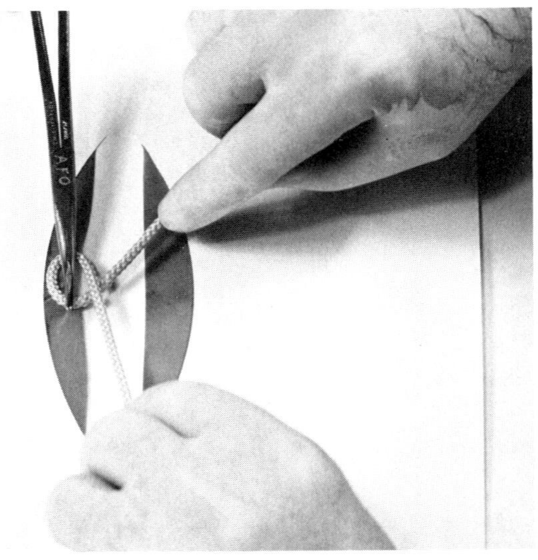

Figure 114. The uncrossed hands hold the crossed ligature.

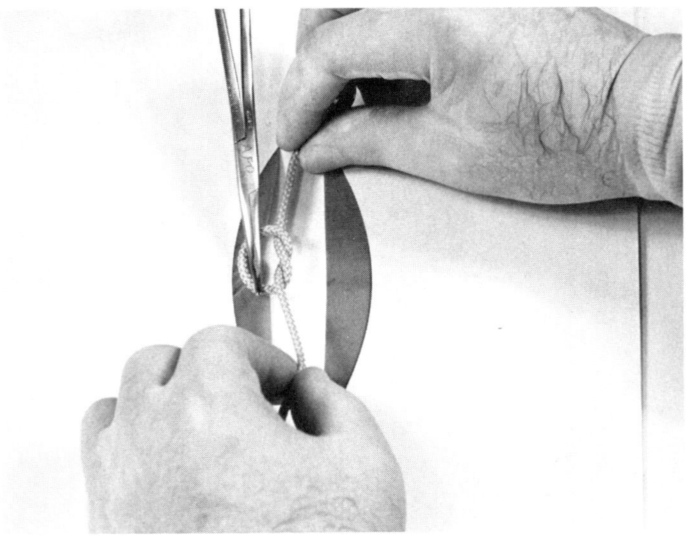

Figure 115. The first half hitch placed flat by the cross technique is in full view for clamp removal.

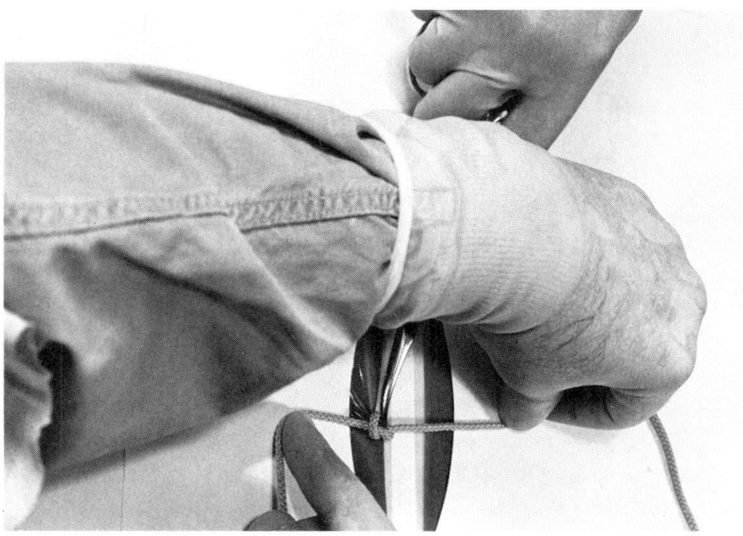

Figure 116. With the uncrossed method, crossing the hands for flat placement of the first half hitch hides the field from the assistant during clamp removal.

With the uncrossed method, crossing hands for flat placement of the first half hitch hides the field from the assistant (Fig. 116), eliminating his visual coordination in clamp removal. An alternative to the uncrossed method allows the assistant to see the knot, but places it in a nonflat attitude.

While passing the tie around the clamp using the crossed method, the free segment may be brought below the fixed one instead of above it. To bring the free end below, it is necessary to grasp with the hand pronated as in Figure 117. Such a hand position occupies more space behind the hemostat than the supinated position shown in Figure 111 and there is greater likelihood of bumping and dislodging the clamp with the right index metacarpal-phalangeal joint.

Step 2.

Trap the encircling loop beneath the tip of the clamp (Fig. 114), then form a half hitch on the sides of the jaws (Fig. 115) with the hands working toward the handles rather than toward the tip, to prevent

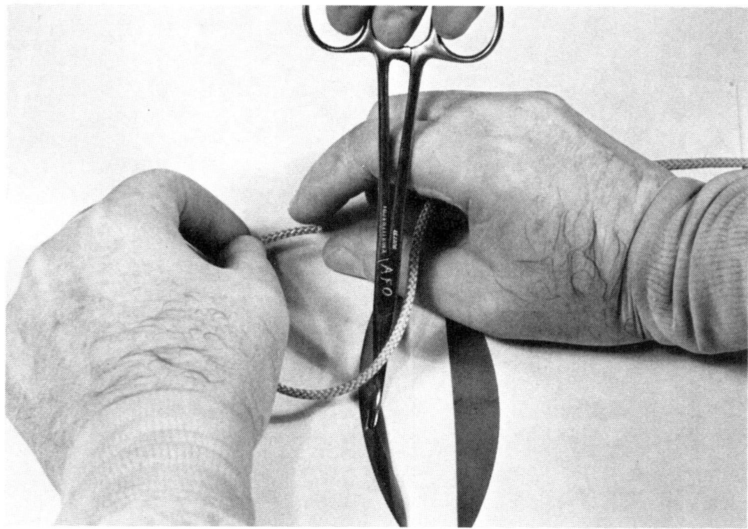

Figure 117. In the crossed method, pressing the free segment below the fixed one has the disadvantage that the clamp may be dislodged when the right hand reaches for the lower free segment.

dislodgment of the trapped suture. Trapping the suture before tying is particularly applicable in deep wounds where the clamp tip is inaccessible for two-handed maneuvering of the half hitch. Also, tying on the sides of the hemostat jaws encasing a wide bite evenly distributes the pressure of the ligature compared to the knot tied off of the tip, thereby reducing the possibility of losing tissue as the clamp is removed.

(Alternate Method)

An alternative Step 2 is to form a half hitch without encircling the tip of the clamp; then place the half hitch beneath the hemostat tip as you tighten the knot. This method avoids the time spent in regular Step 2 and works in noncritical situations where both hands have good access to the wound. A disadvantage lies in the difficulty of sliding a half hitch into a deep wound without stressing the tissue in the clamp.

A half hitch around the shanks acts as a fulcrum between the finger rings and the tip, forming a lever that can tear tissue.

Step 3.

Tighten the knot so as to lay it flat, with the two segments forming a straight angle with each other (Fig. 115). An obtuse angle between the two segments, or failure to balance opposing tensions on the two segments, will stress the tissue, with the hazard of tearing. Placing the tie close to the clamp jaws before tightening the ligature will lessen the amount of devitalized tissue distal to the tie. Spending time to allow the first half hitch to indent the tissue will make the knot more secure than tying with greater pressure while taking less time.

Step 4.

Hold the ligature ends for cutting so that access is provided for the scissor blades, and an adequate view of the knot for the cutter. Discard the cut ends of ligature to leave the field uncluttered.

LIGATURE PASSING, OR "TIE ON A PASSER"

A tie on a passer is a suture held in the jaw tips of a clamp. Ties on passers are used to place ligatures around hemostats on cut vessels in deep wounds. They are also used to pass ties around pedicles which are to be tied in continuity before transection.

Steps in Tying Around a Hemostat

Step 1.

Pass the tip of the passer clamp beyond the hemostat holding the vessel, and hook the ligature with the index finger of your other hand (Fig. 118). Pull the ligature around the hemostat, letting the ligature

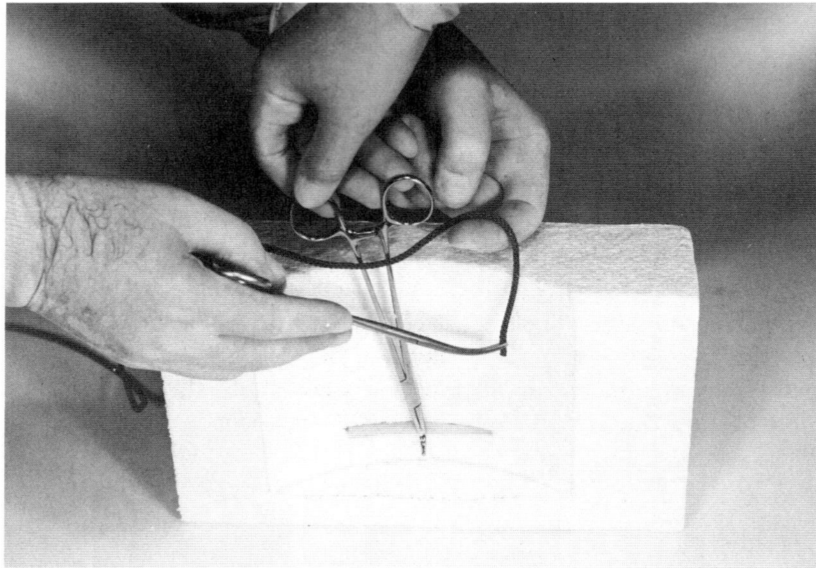

Figure 118. Passing the left hand around the clamp to hook the free end of the ligature.

slide through your hand toward the free end. Avoid the awkward method of passing the passer around the hemostat; the bulk of the clamp being passed is much greater than the bulk of the free end of the tie. Passing the less bulky ligature creates less likelihood of stress and tearing of the clamped tissue.

The principle of the tie on a pass is not to make it more difficult to pass the tie.

Step 2.

Place the ligature around the tip of the hemostat with the passer allowing the tip of the hemostat to trap the ligature (Fig. 119). Maintain enough tension on both segments of the ligature during the remainder of the manipulation to avoid losing the entrapment.

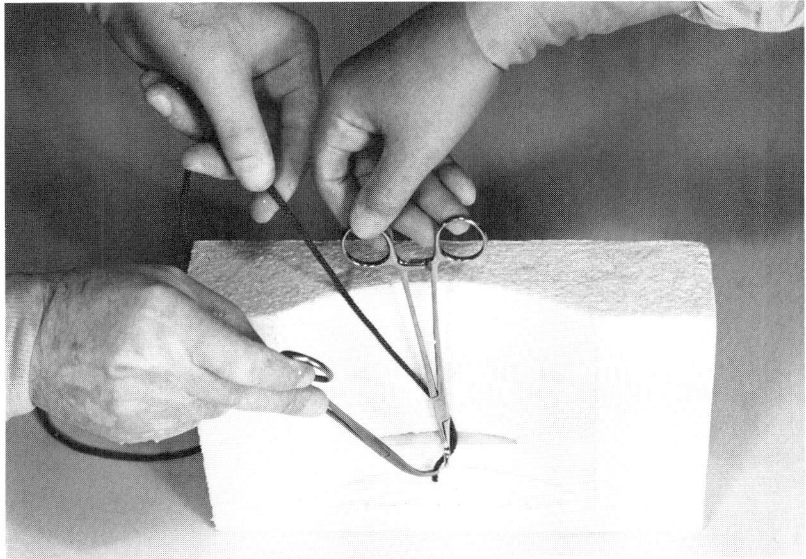

Figure 119. In Step 2 of passing, the ligature is placed so that the tip of the hemostat traps the ligature.

Step 3.

Pull the passer with its segment out of the wound far enough to allow optimal lengths of the two segments for tying (Fig. 120), then remove the passer.

Step 4.

While tying the first half hitch, maintain as much tension on the ligature segments as there is counterpressure on the hemostat, to secure entrapment while forming the half hitch.

Step 5.

Tighten the half hitch with one hand outside the wound while the other maintains tension on its segment with an index finger deep to the knot (Fig. 121). You should gain facility in using either hand within the

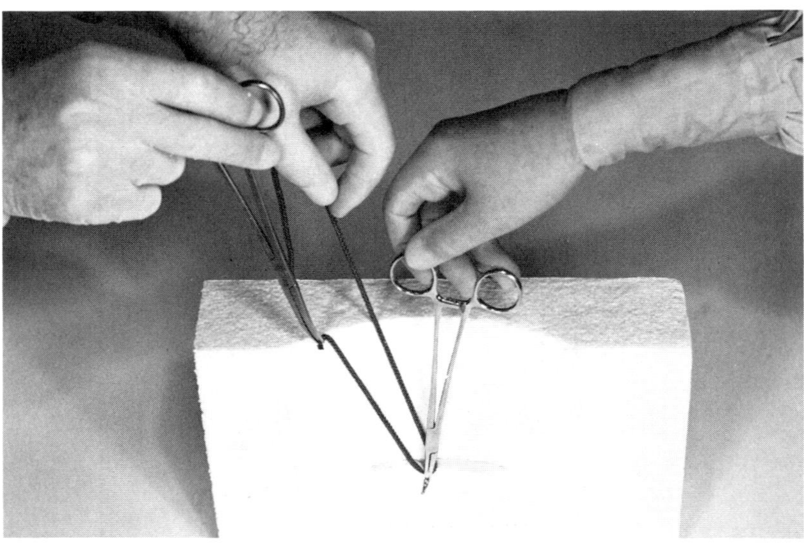

Figure 120. In Step 3, the passer pulls its segment to an adequate length for tying to the other segment.

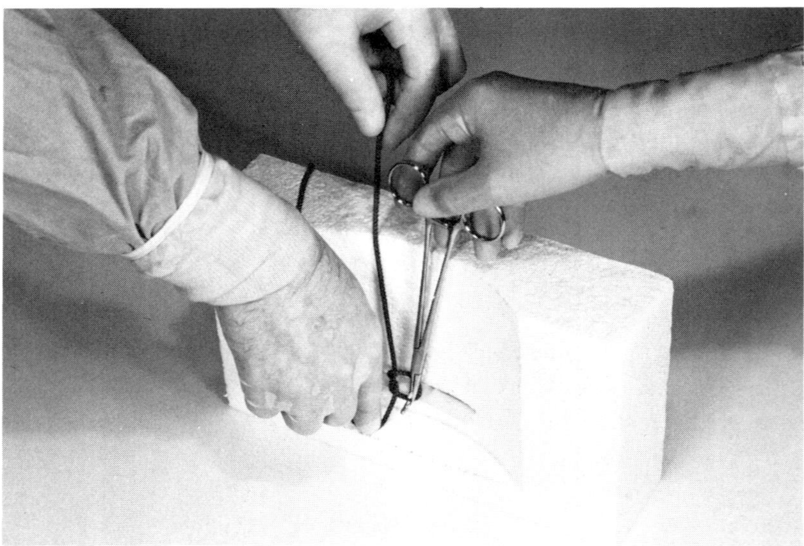

Figure 121. While one hand outside the wound tightens the half hitch, the index finger of the other hand keeps tension on its segment below the knot.

wound, since access to the knot will be on the right in some situations and on the left in others. As the knot is tightened, the tension on one suture should be transferred in a straight line to the other, leaving no tension on the wound except for the tissue within the tie.

Tying Pedicles Before Transection

Tying a pedicle to be transected between ligatures is facilitated by using ties on passers, and can be performed efficiently by the following method.

Step 1.

The surgeon places an angled clamp beneath the pedicle and opens the jaws after it emerges on the other side of the tissue. The assistant then places a tie on a passer, held taut between the free end in one hand and the clamp in the other, deep to the angled clamp's jaws. The surgeon grasps the taut portion of ligature (Fig. 122) with

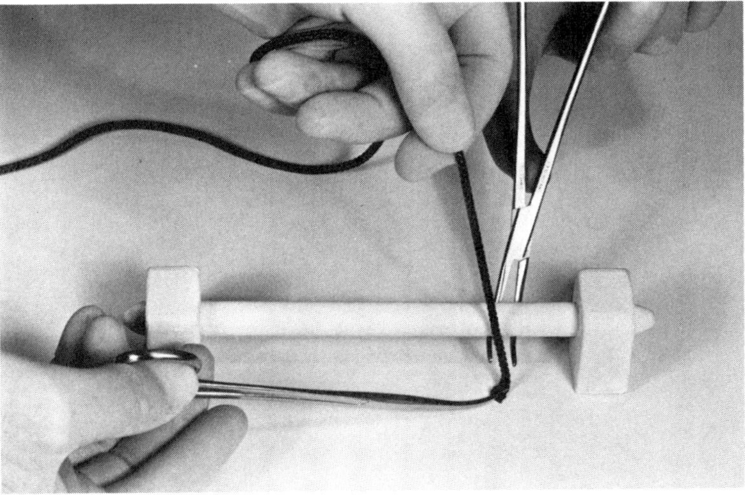

Figure 122. In Step 1 of tying a pedicle before transection, the surgeon maintains control by grasping the taut portion of the ligature with the angled clamp.

the angled clamp. By grasping a taut segment, instead of a free end dangling below the passer, the operators maintain control of the ligature.

Step 2.

The surgeon pauses until he sees that the ligature has been released, before pulling it through. Clamping and pulling the ligature in one motion before it has been released results in a torn pedicle that proves both embarrassing to operators and hazardous to the patient.

Clamping and pulling a ligature as a single motion can cause tears, and tears.

Step 3.

The surgeon takes the free ends in one hand, leaving the assistant with both hands free to pass the second ligature into the reinserted angled clamp's jaws (Fig. 123).

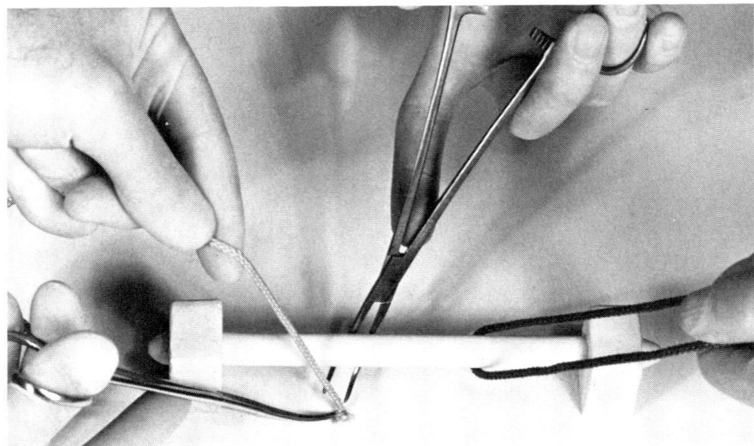

Figure 123. In Step 3 of pedicle tying, the surgeon takes the free ends in one hand, leaving the assistant two free hands to pass the second ligature into the reinserted clamp's jaws.

Step 4.

The assistant retains the second ligature and ties his side first.

Slight retraction in the appropriate direction of one ligature will help maintain distance between the two while the other is tied. Countertraction during tying of one ligature can sometimes be aided by grasping the opposite ligature deep in the wound with an instrument and appropriately directing its tension.

To assure adequate distance between the two ties, the knot tier forms the first half hitch, then before tying it down, places his two index fingers inside the loop (Fig. 124). He then positions the deep portion of the loop against the deep side of the pedicle at the appropriate place, and completes the tie (Fig. 125). As in vessel ligation with a passer, crossing the segments before tying the first half hitch facilitates flat application, with best visibility for both assistant and tier.

CONTROL OF HEMORRHAGE

It is psychologically important for a surgeon to accept the concept totally that the arterial system is a low-pressure hydraulic system.

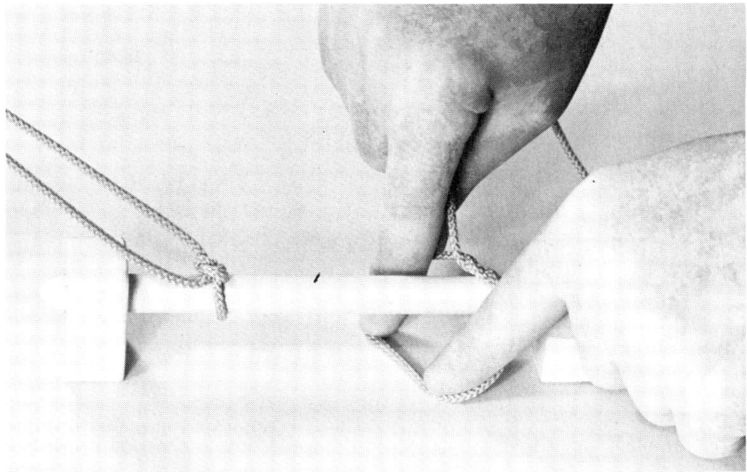

Figure 124. In Step 4 of pedicle tying, to assure adequate distance between the two ties, before tying down the first half hitch, the knot tier places his two index fingers inside the loop below the pedicle.

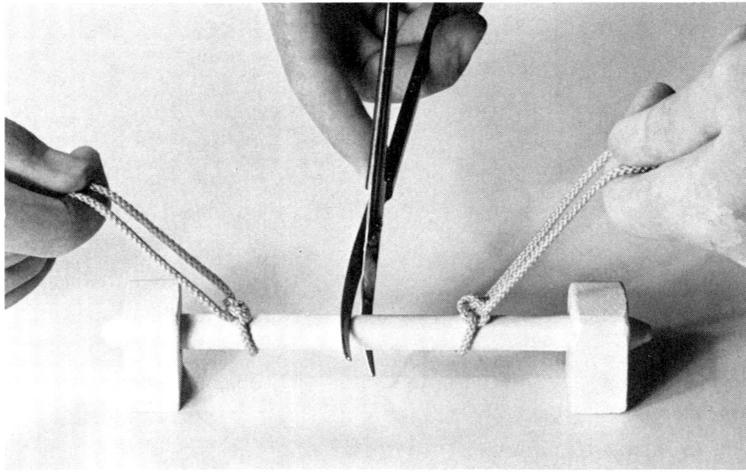

Figure 125. Step 4 is finished by positioning the deep portion of the loop against the deep side of the pedicle and completing the tie.

Such a conviction will prevent him from overreacting to hemorrhage and increase his confidence and ability to manage bleeding.

Hysteria is not a useful adjunct for control of hemorrhage.

The fact that the arterial system is a low-pressure system is demonstrated easily by comparing aortic pressure to that of normal city water supply. The pressure in city water pipes is approximately 45 pounds per square inch (p.s.i.), yet with thumb pressure alone you can easily stop water flowing from a hose. When you consider that normal pressure in the arterial system, by comparison, is only 3 p.s.i., it's quite obvious that you can control bleeding in any major vessel with very gentle pressure. A heavy hand applying enough pressure to stop a 45 p.s.i. hose when placed on a 1½ p.s.i. bleeder may further lacerate the vessel and cause more difficulty instead of solving the problem.

To control massive hemorrhage:

1. Put a finger on the bleeding point and exert the minimal pressure required to stop the bleeding. While one finger controls the bleeding, take time to analyze the situation and make prepara-

tions for definitive control of the hemorrhage. There is no place for frenzy and hurry at this time, as finger pressure control of the bleeding can be maintained for many hours, if necessary.

If the proverbial Dutch boy had had a hemostat, he probably would have made the dike hole larger trying to clamp it off, and Holland would have been flooded.

---

2. Improve the exposure. Placing vascular or other clamps deep within a hole to control major bleeding may damage surrounding structures, resulting in inaccurate placement of clamps or further laceration of blood vessels. You can improve exposure with proximal and distal dissection along the bleeding vessel several centimeters away from the bleeding point.
3. Clamp the bleeding vessel on each side of the bleeding point and remove the hemostatic finger.
4. Repair or ligate the involved vessel.

SURGICAL CLAMPS AS BLUNT DISSECTORS

The smooth tip clamp is a useful instrument for blunt dissection, as it can be used as a probe, as a rake, or as a spreader. A variety of tip angles are applicable to specific uses. Clamps augment the use of dissecting scissors, but, unlike scissors, they slow progress when there is need to alternate frequently between blunt and sharp dissection. Clamps are best used for blunt dissection around vessels and other structures; they can be used alternately for passing ligatures or tapes without the need of changing instruments. Clamps and scissors can be used in concert by two operators. One dissects bluntly with the clamp, while the other cuts the tissue held above the clamp's spread jaws (Fig. 126).

CLAMPS AS TISSUE HOLDERS

Clamps can hold tissue securely over a prolonged period, where static use of tissue forceps would cause fatigue. For example, Kocher

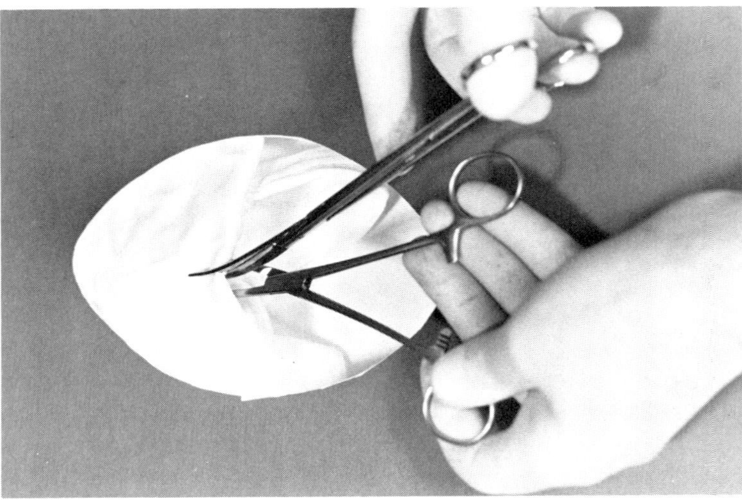

Figure 126. One operator can dissect bluntly with a clamp, while the other operator simultaneously uses scissors to cut tissue above the clamp's spread jaws.

clamps placed on the peritoneal edges will help expose underlying surfaces during separation of adhesions. It is useful to apply a clamp to a gallbladder to stabilize as well as adjust its position during dissection. The selection of clamps is based on the fragility of tissue and the amount of traction needed. Kocher and Allis clamps, with small jaws which apply great pressure to a small area, are applicable for use on fascia but would be traumatic to bowel or lung, where Babcocks or lung clamps can prevent tearing or crushing (Fig. 127).

Atraumatic Clamps. Atraumatic clamps, such as vascular clamps, are designed to hold while exerting the least possible crushing force. Most vascular clamps have fine teeth, so that even with minimal pressure the jaws will not slip off the vessel. The fine teeth exerting pressure on a small portion of the circumference leaves most of the wall between the teeth under no crushing pressure at all (Fig. 128). Vascular clamps are best used when the operator has his own familiar instruments. He can know the holding power at each notch of the ratchets. He can then apply the clamp with the least pressure that

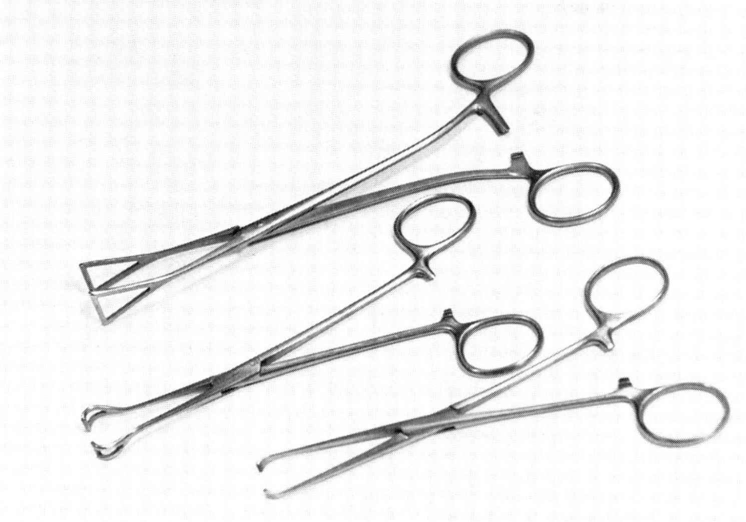

Figure 127.　Duval, Babcock, and Allis clamps.

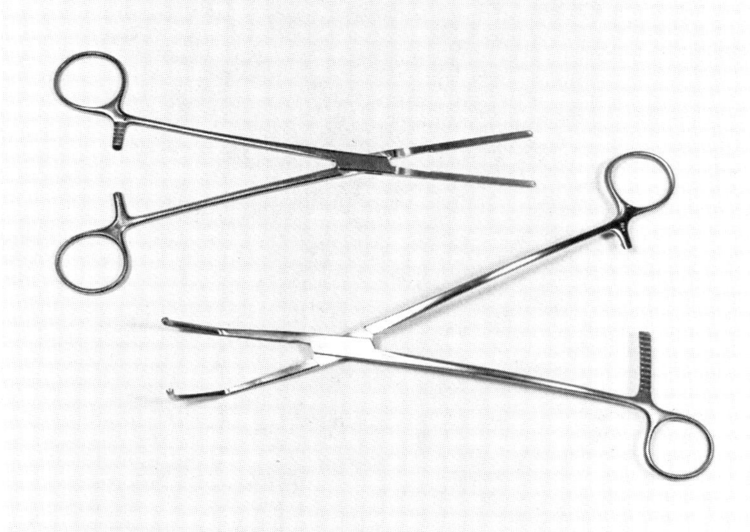

Figure 128.　Vascular clamps are designed, as a rule, with fine teeth, which hold vessels without crushing pressure.

will produce security, thereby minimizing the crushing or cutting of a vessel wall.

Crushing Clamps

Crushing clamps, such as Payrs or large Kochers, used during transection of pedicles or bowel are more secure from having tissue slip between their jaws if a cuff of tissue is left distal to the clamp (Fig. 129). Such an uncrushed cuff is too thick to slip between the jaws. The extra tissue can be excised after the clamp is removed and when it is no longer needed for occlusion or manipulation.

SUMMARY

Hemostasis can be secured with a clamp in two ways: by applying the tip of the bleeding vessel, or by trapping the bleeding vessel in the convexity of its jaws. The tip method leaves a minimum of devitalized

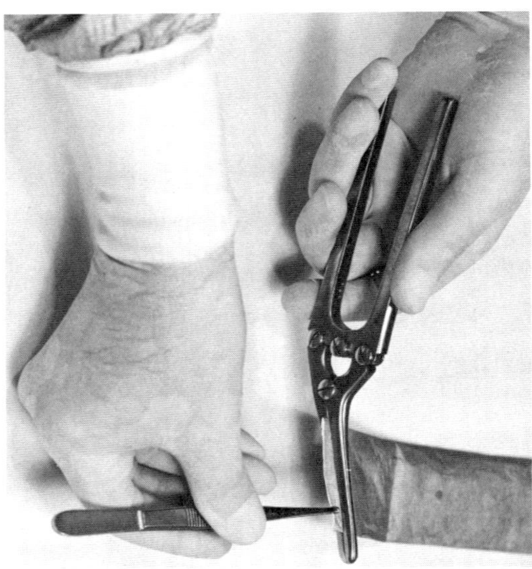

Figure 129. Tissue is not likely to slip from a crushing clamp if a cuff of tissue protrudes distal to the clamp.

tissue in the wound, whereas the jaw technique provides a protruding tip to trap the ligature easily. When clamping a pedicle to be transected, placing the clamps with their tips aimed toward one another leaves the tips in position for holding the suture around the tissue.

Holding the hemostat with a three-point grip provides greater accuracy and security during unclamping. Several clamps can be palmed in the clamping hand if the exposure is good and the situation is noncritical.

When maneuvering the clamp which holds a vessel to be tied, first hold the clamp away from the tissue, then lower it almost parallel to the tissue after the ligature has been placed. Trap the back of the encircling ligature by pushing the tip away from the half hitch being thrown. When tying off the tip, maneuver the clamp to provide the surgeon with the best exposure of the tip. As the first half hitch is tightened, gradually open the clamp to prevent the tissue from escaping out of the ligature.

In noncritical situations, clamps can be held without inserting fingertips through the rings, thus allowing greatest mobility during positioning and removal. A palmed clamp is easier to discard than a clamp held with fingers in the rings.

Clamps are used in blunt dissection by probing between layers of tissue, spreading the jaws within tissue, or by raking tissue aside to expose underlying structures.

Since clamps can hold tissue securely, they are very effective retracting instruments, useful in moving layers of tissue or in maneuvering a mass to allow dissection around it. A spread clamp can be used to elevate a layer of tissue to be transected while protecting structures deep to the dissection.

Clamps function to occlude, grip, dissect, and retract; they become convenient handles for whatever structure they hold within their jaws.

Chapter 7

Electrocautery

Electrocautery techniques used today are refinements of the ancient practice of searing a wound to stop bleeding. The electrocautery current has an alternating sine wave configuration at a radio frequency of approximately 20,000 cycles per second. The cutting mode is a continuous current. The coagulation mode has intermittent, very short bursts of current with relatively long gaps between the bursts.

A continuous current produces more intense heat, which explodes the water to steam in the cells next to the cautery tip, parting them before any significant heat can penetrate to deeper tissue. The cutting current, therefore, leaves a very shallow layer of devitalized, desiccated tissue on the cut surface.

The intermittent coagulation current heats more slowly, causing gradual loss of cellular water, without any steam tearing the tissue apart. Tissue is charred, therefore, rather than divided. The resulting desiccation causes hemostasis by occluding small vessels with coagulated blood and tissue.

Tissue can be cut with the fulgurating current by sustaining the heating until enough charring occurs to disintegrate the tissue. Some cautery units have a blend switch which adds a 120-Hz ripple on the output power supply. The resulting rise and fall in the cutting current increases its charring effect.

Cautery units come with unipolar or bipolar electrodes. The unipolar electrode requires a ground plate placed in contact with the patient. The unipolar electrode is the one most commonly used in surgery. It can both cut and fulgurate.

The bipolar electrode does not require a patient ground plate. Bipolar electrodes usually come in the form of forceps whose tips act as electrodes, allowing the passage of current through tissue when the tips are held about a millimeter apart. The bipolar instrument is a poor cutting tool; the current flows between the electrode tips, not between the electrode and the grounded patient. The bipolar instrument with the current passing directly between the tips is a more effective cautery instrument than the unipolar electrode in a wet field, where current may take a very broad area of least resistance to the indifferent electrode. Bipolar cautery is most commonly used in plastic and neurosurgery, where precise desiccation of small vessels is desired.

The unipolar cautery unit finds many special uses in surgery. The coagulation current is ideal for incising periosteum along a rib or sternum during entry into the chest. A snare cautery is effective in the removal of polyps through a sigmoidoscope. A cutting cautery loop is used by urologists to do prostatic and bladder tumor resections through cystoscopes. Cautery can be used during laparoscopy to fulgurate fallopian tubes for sterilization, during gastroscopy to fulgurate intergastric vessels, and during bronchoscopy for hemostasis after biopsy.

Technique of Application

The single electrode handle can be held in a modified pencil grip between the thumb, middle, and ring fingertips (Fig. 130). Such a grip leaves the index finger free as a "trigger finger," while maintaining a secure grip on the handle. Coagulation is done with the tip of the instrument perpendicular to the wound (Fig. 131). Such a position intensifies the energy to a small area and thus prevents injury to surrounding tissues, as might occur when the side of the tip is in contact with tissue (Fig. 132). Cutting is done with the tip rather than

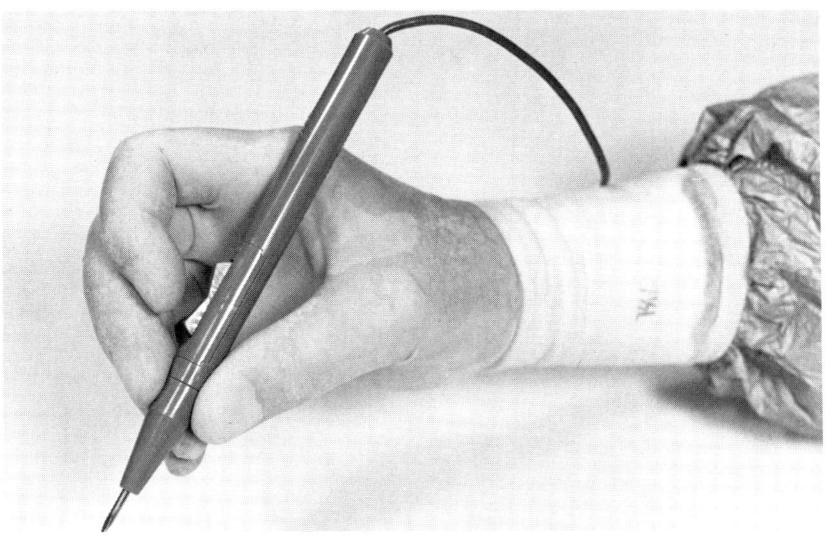

Figure 130. The single electrode cautery handle, held in a modified pencil grip between thumb, middle, and ring fingertips, frees the index "trigger finger."

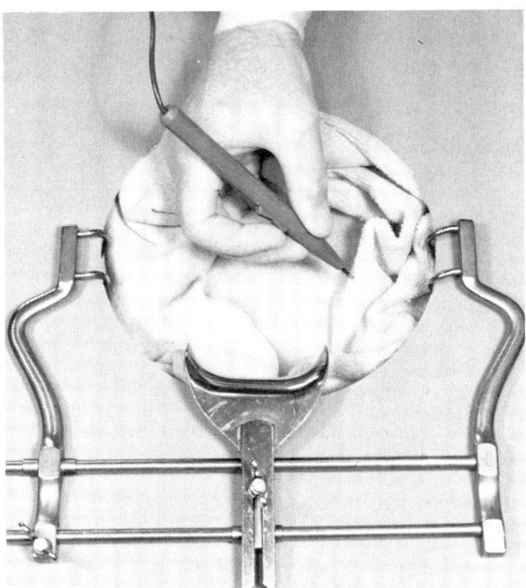

Figure 131. Coagulation is done precisely with the tip of the cautery perpendicular to the wound.

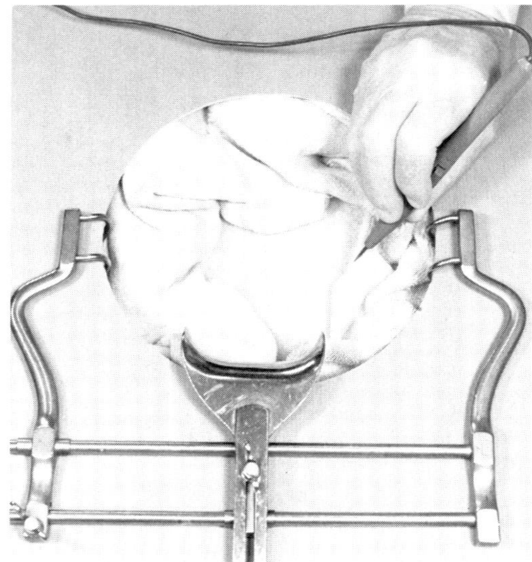

Figure 132. If the side of the cautery tip is applied, tissue not intended for cautery is injured.

the edge of the electrode to localize energy and thus better control the incision. It is important to clean the cautery tip frequently to prevent a buildup of char which would disperse the current to a larger area of tissue, thereby diminishing the control.

If you use your trigger finger to hold your gun, you may fire it accidentally.

With a unipolar electrode, the drier the wound the more localized the current, and the more effective the coagulation. Coagulation of blood vessels is more efficient with good coordination of assistants and the surgeon in maintaining a dry field by pressure control of bleeding points and effective removal of blood by sponging and sucking. There are some situations where pressure near the bleeding sites will give enough control to allow effective cautery. If bleeding is brisk, the most satisfactory coagulation for hemostasis is obtained by clamping the open end of the vessel, then running the cautery current through the clamp by touching the clamp with the cautery tip. For large bleeders, clamping and tying is more secure.

Trying to cauterize in a pool of blood with a unipolar tip is both ineffective and frustrating.

Where depth control is critical in the use of electrocautery near such vital structures as large vessels, bowel, and nerve, using the open end of a clamp to elevate the layer to be cut will protect such underlying structures (Fig. 133). Another protective method is to interpose an insulating object between the vital structure and the cautery. A tongue blade inserted between the heart and the pericardial sac will allow opening of the sac using cautery without hazard to the coronary vessels (Fig. 134). Avoid touching the skin with the coagulating current; small unsightly third degree burns may result.

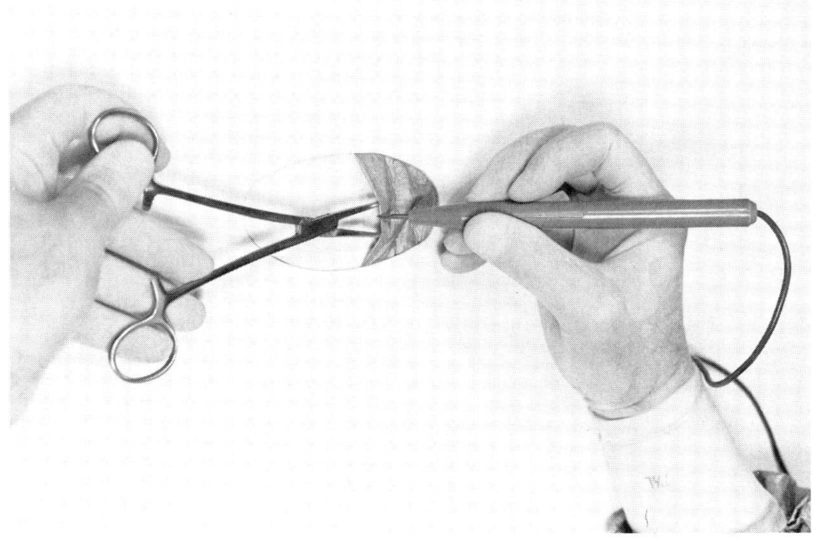

Figure 133. Using the open end of a clamp to elevate a layer to be cut by cautery will protect vital underlying tissues.

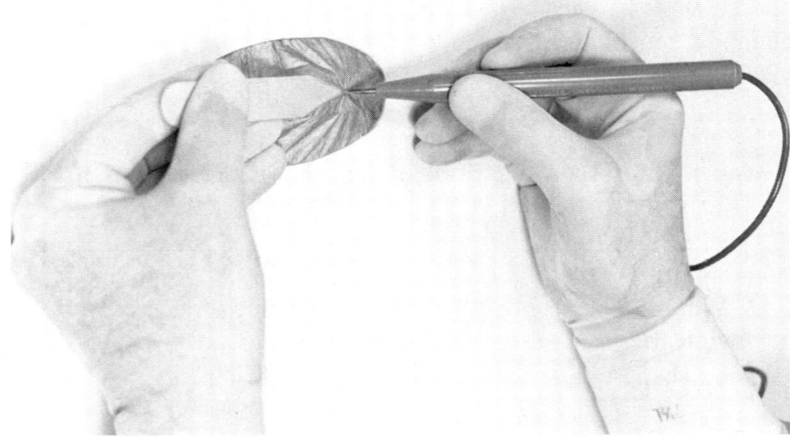

Figure 134. An insulating tongue blade interposed between heart and pericardial sac allows cutting of the sac by cautery, without risk to coronary vessels.

If you use an electrocautery when you have a hole in your glove you will have vividly demonstrated what damage the cautery can do to the skin.

After the epidermis has been incised with a scalpel, the dermis may be cut with a cutting current without untoward effects on the ultimate scar and with the benefit of coagulating the rich vascular plexus in the subdermis.

When cutting muscle with electrocautery, the current should be allowed to do the cutting without exerting undue pressure on the tissue with the instrument. Progress should be slow enough that vessels are coagulated before severing, to prevent retraction of the vessel into the muscle mass. If a vessel is seen to cross the proposed incision, blood is saved by fulgurating the vessel on either side before the incision is made. The coagulation cautery, being more hemostatic than the cutting mode, is safer to use for cutting on a patient with a coagulopathy, where slight increase in char within the wound is an acceptable trade for prevention of bleeding. Electrocautery can be used to coagulate small vessels near vital structures if the setting is turned to very low power. Desiccation of vasa brava of the aorta can be a safe procedure with the appropriate power setting of the electrosurgical unit.

Let the electric current do the cutting. Trying to cut with pressure will decrease depth control.

These are two special requirements for use of bipolar electrodes (Fig. 135): there must be continuity of electrolyte fluid (water, electrolytes, and tissue) between the tips, or current will not be conducted and coagulation will not occur; there must be a gap between the two tips; if

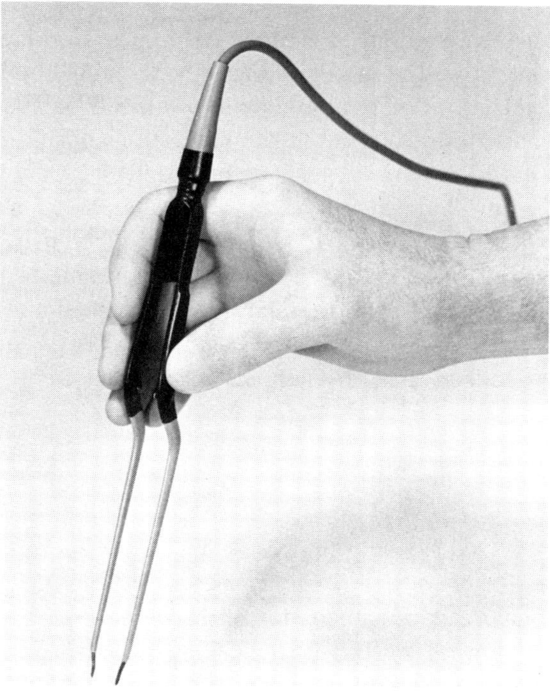

Figure 135. For effectual use of bipolar electrodes there must be a gap between the tips to prevent short circuit, and there must be continuity of conducting electrolyte fluid between the tips.

the tips touch one another the current will "short" between them without generating adequate heat for desiccation. Lack of understanding of these two requirements has caused frustration during the early experience of many surgeons.

A charring aortotomy is not yet a recognized form of entry, though it may score a few points with your patient's lawyer.

Advantages and Disadvantages of Electrocautery

The advantages of electrocautery can be summed up in economy of blood loss, a drier field, and speed.

The main disadvantage in cautery lies in poor depth control. Cutting or coagulating with a cautery can easily damage underlying structures. A cauterized vessel is more liable to rebleed because of dislodgment of a coagulum from the trauma of the continuing surgery, whereas a ligated vessel is permanently and securely obliterated. Cautery has no mechanical feel of tissue tension, such as the grain of the tissue or definition of layers, as can be felt when using scissors or scalpel. Cautery used to transect muscle can stimulate contractions that distort and detract from the accuracy of transection. The cautery, if improperly used, can deter wound healing by leaving an inordinate amount of devitalized tissue within the wound.

Hazards of Cautery

A cautery used casually can result in severe unintentional burns. Towel clips used to fasten the cautery wire to the operative field have, on occasion, perforated the insulation of the wire, causing third-degree burns. Inadvertent triggering of the switch with the cautery tip lying next to the patient or against any instrument in the field results in an unplanned burn.

Explosions with electrocautery have come from two sources. The explosion of anesthetic gases is less likely with the advent of less hazardous anesthetic agents. The hazard of explosion of gas within the bowel is ever present when cauterizing through a sigmoidoscope or when opening the bowel with a cutting current. In these situations it is important to evacuate the bowel gas and exchange it with air before use of the cautery.

Experience may not be the best teacher, but it is frequently the most dramatic.

The hazard of accidentally using the undesired mode of current or having the cautery accidentally on is minimized by having a sound that is audible when the instrument is running, with different characteristic tones for cutting and coagulation.

In summary, the electrocautery is an indispensable surgical instrument that materially contributes to reduction of blood loss and the efficiency of operation.

Chapter 8

Tools for Providing Exposure

One of the basic secrets of good surgery is good exposure. Many students who perform their first operation find it very easy with an expert teacher as an assistant. Then, when the student tries the same procedure for the first time with a student assistant whose experience is less than his, he finds the operation very difficult. Exposure and retraction in the first situation were planned and maintained by the teacher, and unnoticed by the novice until, with the less experienced assistant, he had to produce the exposure for himself.

Even though the retractor is the first tool to which the student is introduced in the operating room, it is probably the last one that he masters in his metamorphosis to a surgeon. It takes planning and good execution to establish good exposure. The surgeon should accomplish the exposure by placing the packing sponges and the retractors. It is a mistake to leave to an assistant a facet of an operation as important as exposure, and then regard him as a poor assistant if he fails to obtain good exposure for you.

If an operation was difficult for you, your exposure was poorly planned.

Stabilizing the Exposure
(Sponges, Bags, Tapes, and Stitches)

The first consideration in the use of exposure tools is stabilizing mobile structures that tend to creep into the field by gravity, elasticity, or respiratory movements. Stabilization provides a field that does not require repeated time-consuming readjustments of the exposure.

A sponge placed over slippery structures allows retraction of them as though they were a single unit. The friction of the coarse sponge fibers grips slippery tissue, reducing the possible motion of the structures. Sponges are more inclined to stay in place if they are wrapped around structures in such a way that tissue cannot outflank the sponge (Fig. 136). If the sponge can be positioned beneath and

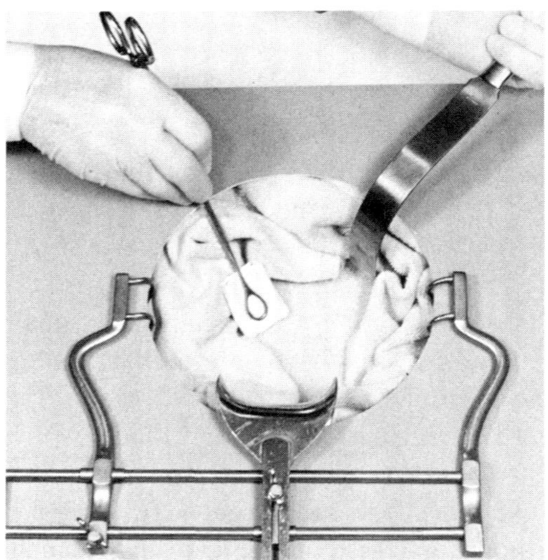

Figure 136. Sponges should be placed beneath and around the area needing stabilized exposure. The self-retaining retractor shown is the Balfour. Upper right shows a hand retractor. Right hand holds a stick sponge.

around adjoining sides of an area to be exposed, there is better chance of sustained exposure than if the structure to be retracted is merely covered where visibility is needed.

Stitches placed on edges of peritoneum, pleura, or dura, then folded back over sponges, help stabilize the sponge exposure (Fig. 137). Structures will then stay put, as the sponges will not ride up, exposing tissue between the serous edge and a retractor.

Plastic bags designed for complete envelopment of intestines allow retraction of this mobile structure as a unit and therefore have great advantage in some applications (Fig. 138). Such plastic bags, as well as improving exposure, have the advantage of preventing drying of the exposed tissue.

Dry sponges cling to tissue more firmly than wet ones and therefore provide more stable exposure, but they have the disadvantage of traumatizing surfaces that may then adhere to one another, forming adhesions during the recovery process. Such adhesions can be a significant disadvantage in the abdomen, but may be of no disadvantage in other wounds, such as in the thoracic cavity, where pleural synthesis

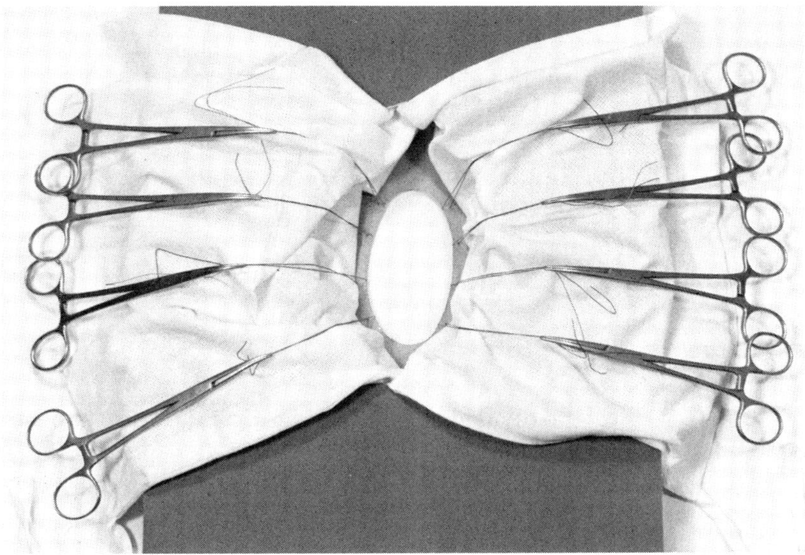

Figure 137. Stitches placed on edges of peritoneum, pleura, or dura, then folded back over sponges, help stabilize the exposure.

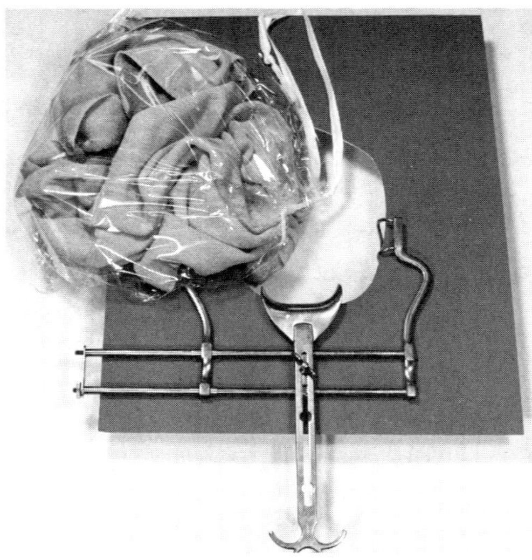

Figure 138. A plastic bag for envelopment and retraction of the intestines can both improve exposure and prevent drying of the retracted structures.

may sometimes be desired. Proper placement of sponges to stabilize tissue allows retractors to be placed securely to provide unchanging exposure of the operative field.

Don't be outflanked by nonstabilized tissue
because of poor packing.

Retractors

Retractors can be divided into two categories: the basic exposure retractors and minor variation retractors. The basic exposure retractors are placed to provide unchanging, long-term retraction of the wound for a major portion of the surgical procedure. These should be self-retaining retractors whenever possible. Self-retaining retractors accomplish nonchanging continuous retraction without causing fatigue in the assistants. They also free hands to help with nonstationary work and rid the field of the clutter of unnecessary retracting hands and arms. Self-retaining retractors allow the surgeon to position the assistants so as not to compromise his access to the field. There are a few situations where an assistant must provide long-term, uninterrupted strong traction. The large variety of available self-retaining retractors ensures that there is one applicable to almost any surgical procedure. Abdominal ring retractors (Fig. 139), Balfour retractors (Fig. 136), rib spreaders, sternal spreaders, Weitlaners (Fig. 140), and spring retractors are a few of the commonly available ones. The major hazard of self-retaining retractors is ischemia at the pressure point. During long procedures it is often wise to release the retraction periodically to prevent devitalization of the wound edges which might result in poor wound healing.

The poorer the exposure planning, the harder the assistant has to pull on the retractor.

Minor variation retractors can be used by assistants to fine tune the exposure, once the basic self-retaining retraction is provided. Be-

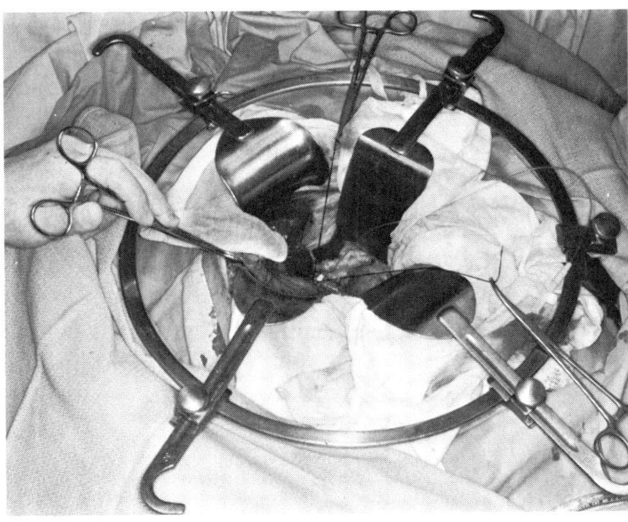

Figure 139. The abdominal ring retractor shown is self-retaining for sustained strong traction.

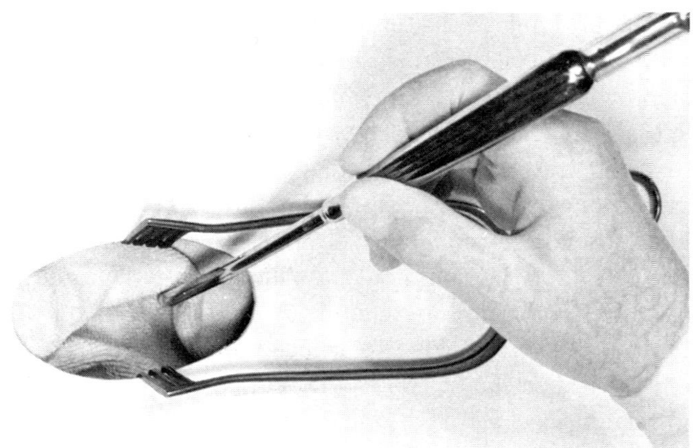

Figure 140. The self-retaining retractor shown is the Weitlaner. The hand holds suction apparatus without compromising visibility and accessibility for the surgeon.

sides hand retractors (Fig. 136), clamps, stick sponges (Fig. 136), peanut sponges, suction apparatus (Fig. 140), and assistants' hands will accomplish needed variations in the fixed exposure.

The hand-held retractor is the tool used by surgeons to minimize competition by discouraging medical students from becoming surgeons.

Adequate exposure requires accessibility as well as visibility. Pulling up on retractors can expose structures but may create such a deep hole as to make the operative site inaccessible. Depressing retractors, on the other hand, can make wounds shallower and structures more accessible. A good example of retraction designed to depress surrounding tissue and deliver the target site is seen with the use of Lange-type retractors. With such a retractor the bone is elevated with the tip while surrounding tissue is pressed downward with the shaft (Fig. 141).

A great hazard in the use of retraction of all types is inadvertent tissue laceration by excessive pull or by using inappropriate retracting tools. Only one person should pull on a retractor at a time. If two

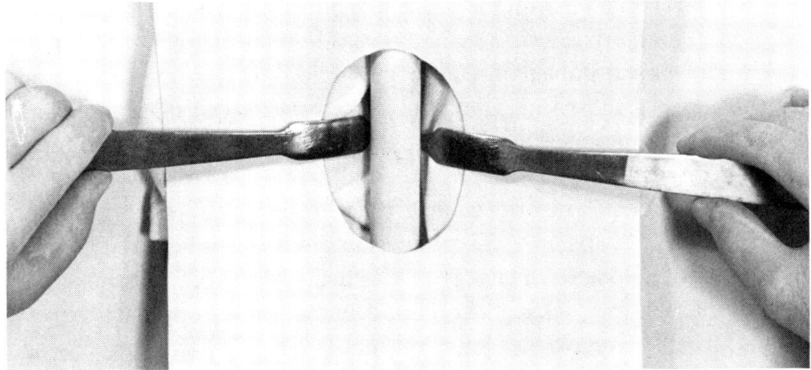

Figure 141. Lange-type retractors, whose tips elevate the bone and whose shafts depress surrounding tissue, provide good accessibility as well as good visibility.

people pull on a retractor, neither can sense the amount of tug applied by the other, so that tissue strength may be inadvertently exceeded. It is, therefore, important for an assistant to release his tension on a retractor whenever the surgeon takes it for repositioning or to manipulate the retractor himself. In retracting fragile structures where lacerations might result from a sharp, rigid edge, the hand placed over a sponge, or a stick sponge, may be superior to a metal retractor.

If you want to tear a liver or lacerate a mesentery, two can pull harder than one.

Traction and Countertraction:
An Aid to Dissection

Accurate secure dissection depends upon continuing exposure and stabilization of the tissue being dissected. Self-retaining and other retractors along with packing sponges provide general field exposure, while the specific field of dissection requires ongoing exposure and stabilization of tissue achieved through progressive traction and countertraction.

Expert surgeons employ the principles of traction and counter-traction in many dissecting maneuvers. Most tissue planes will remain flaccid and closed unless one applies traction away from a fixed (countertracting) structure or movable (countertracting) instrument. This principle becomes useful when dissecting the upper flap of a mastectomy or creating a pouch for a pacemaker.

The surgeon sets up countertraction by placing his assistant's hooks, rakes, clamps or other retraction devices, and exerting traction in a direction opposite to that from the assistant's instrument. He may have his assistant pick up the tissue immediately opposite him with tissue forceps or clamp so he can exert traction away from the assistant's countertraction, thus tensing and spreading the tissue to be divided. As the surgeon dissects along a structure, moving his traction instrument, the assistant may need to move his instrument simultaneously, grasping tissue opposite and applying traction in a counter-direction (Fig. 142).

Directed traction and countertraction keep the operation moving while enhancing the accuracy and security of the dissection.

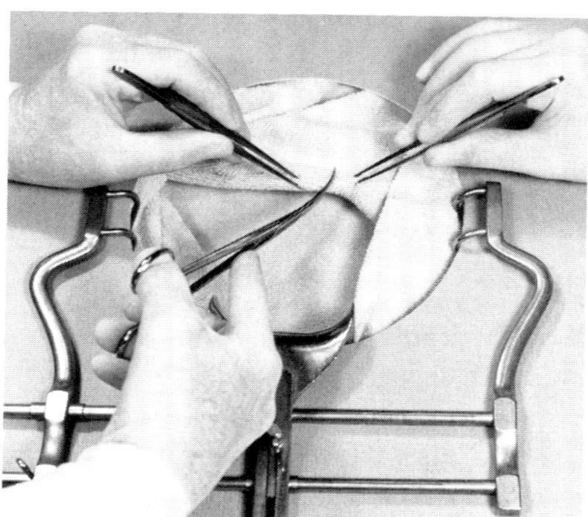

Figure 142. As the surgeon dissects, the surgeon and the assistant simultaneously move their traction instruments to provide consistent traction and countertraction.

A good assistant becomes an invaluable aid in dissection when he masters the principle of countertraction to the point where it becomes automatic. An experienced surgeon sometimes uses countertraction to lead a junior resident through an operation—sometimes with no more than a sponge stick in one hand and a sucker in the other. He exposes the right tissue planes, selecting, then tensing the tissue for the resident to cut.

One difference between the expert and novice surgeon is that the expert directs his dissection toward what is to be left behind; whereas the novice directs his dissection toward what is to be taken out.

Removal of Blood from a Wound
(Use of Suction and Sponges)

Maintaining a dry, bloodless field is paramount to good exposure. Suction and sponging should be performed so as to provide the best exposure with the least interruption of the surgeon's dissection. The sucker tip can be placed just ahead of the dissection in progress, in a manner that does not compromise the surgeon's view while at the same time leaving room for manipulation of his tools (Fig. 140). When intermittently sucking or sponging in synchrony with a surgeon entering and leaving the wound, it is better to synchronize withdrawal of the suction or sponge with the surgeon's entrance into the wound, rather than with his exit. If one enters the wound with a sucker tip as the surgeon removes his tools, then removes the sucker tip after aspirating all of the free blood, blood may reaccumulate before the surgeon is ready to proceed with his work. It is, therefore, best to synchronize withdrawal of the aspirating tip or sponge just as the surgeon enters the wound.

There is some hazard of aspiration injury to tissue from sucker tips with a single terminal opening. A finger hole on the handle of such instruments is usually provided to limit the suction if the terminal opening is occluded against tissue. A concept of covering the finger hole whenever one desires to suck, rather than one of releasing the hole to prevent suction, will "accentuate the positive" and will prevent inadvertent trauma.

A skillfully performed operation can be done only with superior exposure that is well planned, continuously maintained, and rarely accidental.

When aspirating on delicate tissue, the interposition of fabric such as a sponge or cottonoid will allow removal of fluid without the hazard of tissue trauma. Sucker tips should be adequate for the job at hand. There are a variety of sucker tips, from ones with holes large enough to aspirate clots and large amounts of blood, to fine tips.

There is an advantage in aspirating large quantities of blood rather than using sponges for removal, as suction permits keeping a more accurate account of blood loss. Sponges are designed to soak up fluid and are therefore used to blot, not rub or wipe the tissue clean. Rubbing removes clots, abrades tissue, and promotes further bleeding. Stick sponges, besides being useful retractors and useful for sponging blood, can be used to tamponade bleeding in large vessels such as the aorta or iliac arteries by pressing stick sponges firmly against the vessel. Such use of stick sponges will allow hemostasis in emergency situations while dissecting around the vessels to gain security and safety in the application of vascular clamps.

Chapter 9

Operating Room Tools

Surgeons always feel more secure working in the Operating Room than when performing the same procedure in an Emergency Room, Intensive Care Unit, or in an Outpatient Clinic. The security is partly psychological; the Operating Room is his most familiar workshop. However, the security also depends upon having an optimal operating table, superior lighting, and sophisticated monitoring equipment. Security is also provided by personnel who are familiar with the surgeon's methods, who can provide tools and equipment with minimal briefing and without delay.

The O.R. is the surgeon's security blanket.

The surgeon can maximize his security in the operating room if he uses the facilities with control over details in their proper sequence. If not, he will find himself gowned, gloved, and then frustrated by his inability subsequently to correct the improper position of the patient on the operating table, the inappropriate position of monitor and vascular lines, the absence of an indifferent cautery plate, the inadequate lighting, and the absence of critical instruments necessary to do the procedure.

When a surgeon is in the operating room he feels as secure as in his mother's womb.

The Operating Room Table

The proper position of the operating room table allows optimal access for the work of the anesthesiologist, the surgeon, and the instrument technician. Head and neck surgery requires coordination of the needs of the anesthetist and the surgeon to properly position the table with reference to anesthetic equipment.

Ether Screens

A variety of ether screens and tunnels are available; select one that will afford access to the patient for both surgeon and anesthesiologist, without either infringing on the necessary territory of the other. Position the screen so that the risers will not be in the way of the surgical manipulation.

Ether screens are appropriately referred to in some operating rooms as "windshields."

X-Ray Cassette Tunnel

If intraoperative X-rays are to be taken, make certain that the cassette tunnel is positioned in the proper place under the table before draping, so as to provide access for the X-ray technician without need for repositioning during the procedure.

Positioning the Patient

After induction of anesthesia, the surgeon will gain great security by positioning the patient on the operating table himself. Such positioning will avoid the hazard of contaminating the operative field with attempts at alteration after the patient is prepped and draped. The position of the patient should be made secure, using sandbags, straps, tapes, pads, and rests, to prevent shifting during the procedure. An excellent method is the use of "bean bags," from which air can be evacuated after positioning the patient; the result is a formfitting "case" for the patient (Fig. 143).

The table height should be adjusted so that the tallest member of the operating team can stand without the strain of bending and stooping. Other members can stand on appropriate height lifts to give all personnel optimal visibility and functional advantage. The table height that provides for the surgeon's optimal working position is usually with the operative field at the level of the surgeon's elbows (Fig. 144). His elbows are then in midposition between flexion and extension, thereby allowing mobility in all directions.

It is the surgeon's responsibility to check pressure points that

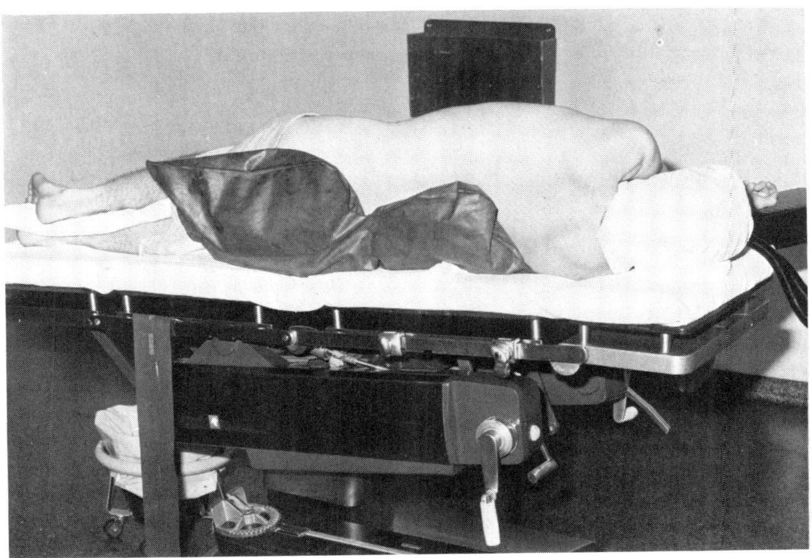

Figure 143. A formfitting case of bean bags positions the patient.

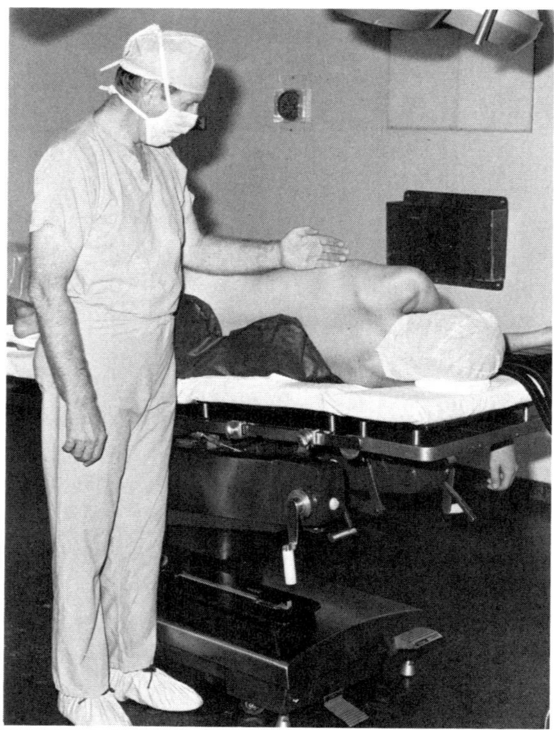

Figure 144. Optimal table height places the operative field at the level of the surgeon's elbows.

need to be protected in order to prevent temporary or permanent injury to the patient. Placement of a soft pad beneath the pressure point may not be adequate to prevent the effects of pressure, because the pad, whether hard or soft, does not relieve the weight on that point. In some cases, padding beneath a pressure point may even increase the hazards of pressure. Instead of padding pressure points, elevate these points by placing pads under surrounding structures; pressure points will then not be in contact with the table. For example, padding beneath the calves, thereby elevating the heels from the table, will prevent pressure on the heels when a patient is in the supine position (Fig. 145). A padded doughnut is far better protection to the base of the skull than a pad beneath the head, as the doughnut completely elevates the inion from the table (Fig. 146).

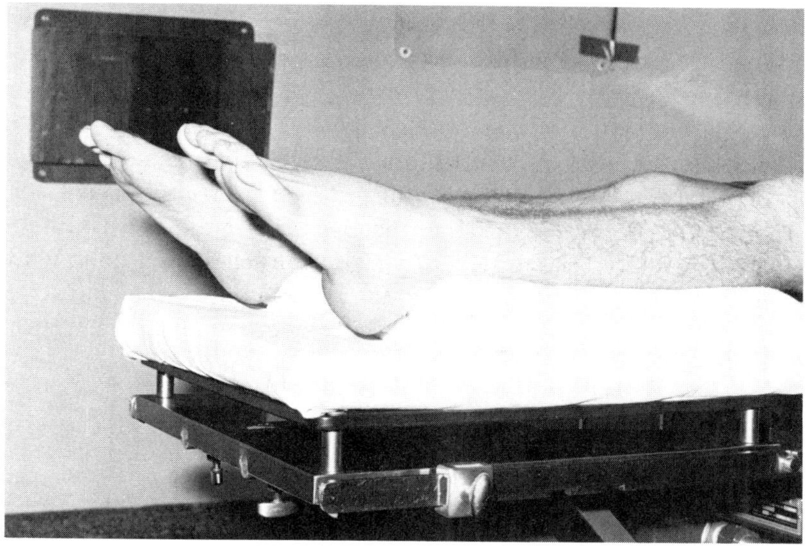

Figure 145. To prevent pressure on the heels, pad the calves of the supine patient.

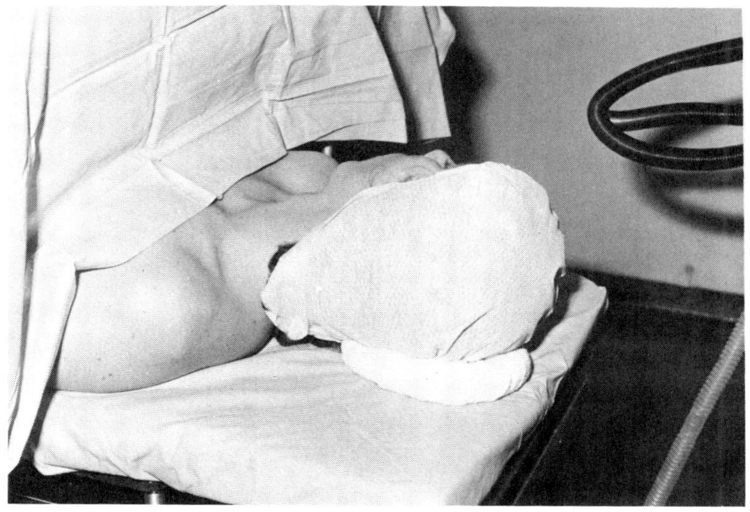

Figure 146. Since a doughnut elevates the inion from the table, it is better protection from pressure on the base of the skull than a pad under the head.

Padding the pressure point increases the pressure on that point.

Check the position of arms to assure that there is no tension on the brachial plexus. Position the arms to provide an optimal compromise between access for the anesthesiologist and access to the operative field for the surgeon. Special attention should be given to places where nerves are vulnerable to pressure injury. The leg straps should not go across the head of the fibula where peroneal nerve pressure may cause temporary or permanent foot drop.

Lines

All intravenous and intra-arterial lines should be taped securely prior to prepping and draping, so that there is no possibility of their kinking during the procedure when they are inaccessible for adjustment. The curve of the tubing as it doubles back should be taped so that it cannot kink if traction is inadvertently applied (Fig. 147). It is extremely important to tape all connections of tubing, particularly arterial, before they are hidden from the view of the anesthesiologist during the procedure. All connections should be Luer-Lok. Hypovole-

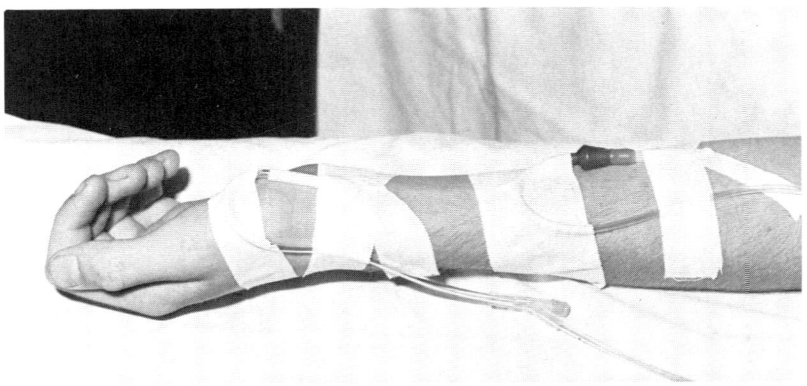

Figure 147. The double-back curve of intravenous tubing should be taped so that it cannot kink.

mia, with subsequent complications, including death, has occurred as a consequence of arterial line connections coming loose in small children, resulting in blood loss hidden from the view of the anesthesiologist and other operating room personnel.

The indifferent cautery electrode, EKG wires, and other monitoring sensors should be secure before the patient is covered with drapes. Many an operation has been compromised by shortcutting details in the securing of lines prior to proceeding with a surgical prep.

Monitoring Equipment

Monitoring a patient not only helps guide the course of his operation, but should be important to subsequent patients by providing data for retrospective analysis and prospective planning of procedures. Data collection, when thoroughly planned, should not be frustrated by careless preparation of recording instruments and their patient connections. Equipment and supplies should be checked before, not during, the operation.

Visual display screens are best placed where the surgeon, anesthetist, and monitor technician can see them without turning away from their work.

Lights

One of the major advantages of an operating room over other environments is the superior lighting. Position these lights for optimal illumination prior to scrubbing. Then make fine adjustments with sterile light handles during the procedure. A wide variety of overhead lights in the past have been a constant bugaboo to surgeons, as the light is always in need of adjustment. Shadows from hands and instruments are intermittently in the way, and deep recesses are difficult to look into, as the surgeon's head invariably eclipses the overhead lights. The recent introduction of coaxial fiberoptic headgear has been a significant improvement. With a beam of parallel light originating from between the surgeon's eyes, any place he focuses his attention is brightly lit, thereby eliminating the need for constant overhead light adjustments. Don't give up if you try a headlight and don't like it at first. Most frustration experienced by surgeons using headlights for the first time comes from inadequate preoperative adjustment of the headband and light focus. If you give it a chance, you will eventually become addicted to the headlight. If a surgeon is wearing a headlight, his assistant should, also. The field will then not become dark if the surgeon looks away while the assistant is finishing a maneuver.

The ability to work well in the dark should be a wasted talent in surgery.

The surgeon's scrub should start only after he has checked the operating table position, the patient's position, pressure points, all lines, cables, and monitoring equipment, and has determined that his light is satisfactory and that essential operating tools are available for the procedure.

A minute check at the proper time saves nine.

Drapes

Drapes are designed to keep a sterile field, but if improperly used can have the opposite effect. A drape can become a wick from nonsterile areas if blood runs down along the drapes to the table. Where a wick effect is anticipated, it can be prevented by sealing a plastic sterile drape to the field and allowing it to drape down past the tabletop. The plastic can then be covered with a cloth or other drape, once there is security against such contamination.

In applying field towels after application of the large operative table drapes, place the side drapes first, then the cephalad and caudad ones will keep the side drapes in place (Fig. 148). On the other hand, if you place the cephalad and caudad ones first, the ends of the side drapes placed last will fall away from the clip fastenings and expose the field the towels should cover (Fig. 149).

In applying wound towels, take care to prevent the operative

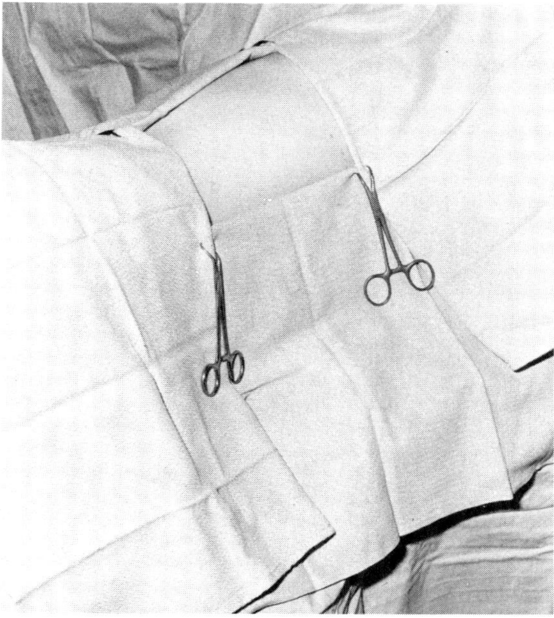

Figure 148.   When side field towels are placed first, the cephalad and caudad towels keep the side drapes in place.

exposure from being limited by the towels. Use a procedure that leaves the skin towels more redundant than the skin. To assure adequate exposure, clip the wound towels at one end of the incision (Fig. 150), then pull on that clip to stretch the skin, then apply a towel clip at the other end of the wound. When the tension is released from the wound clamps at the two ends, the opening between the towels will, therefore, be longer than the incision. The incision can then be stretched when necessary by retractors.

Don't hide the operative field with poorly applied wound towels.

The three methods of fastening wound towels are useful in specific situations. In most major operations the towels are clipped to the skin by towel clips. In more minor procedures, where there is little

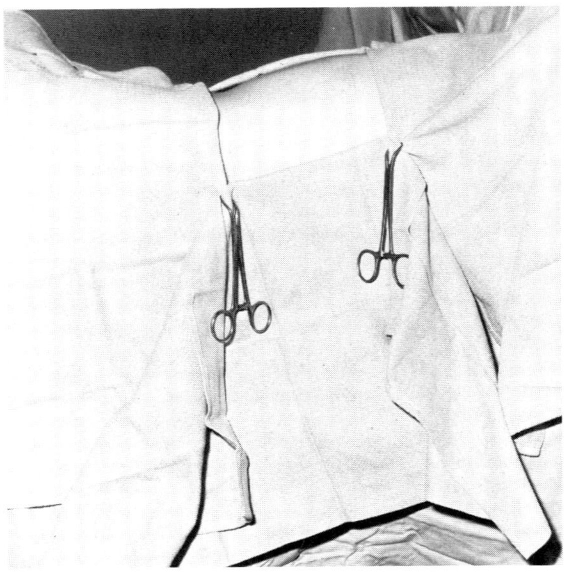

Figure 149. If the cephalad and caudad towels are placed first, the side towels will fall away from the clip fastenings.

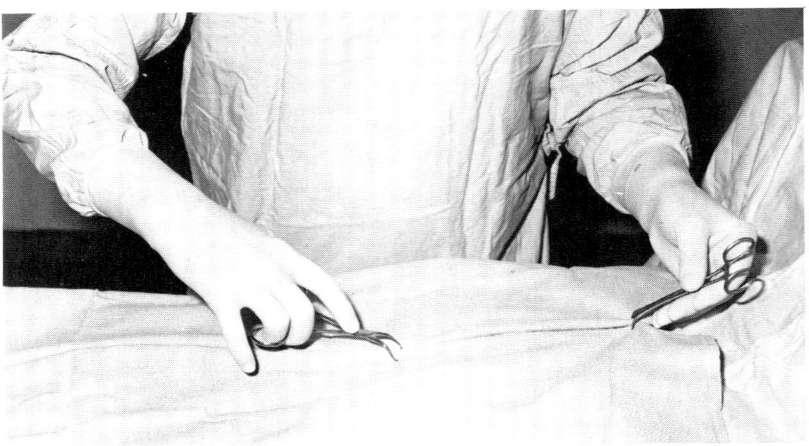

Figure 150. To assure adequate exposure after applying wound towels, clip the towels at one end of the incision, pull on that clip to stretch the skin, then apply a towel clip at the other end of the wound. When tension is released from the wound clamps at the two ends, the opening between the towels will be longer than the exposed skin.

danger of drape slipping during the operation, clips can be fastened merely to the towels and not pierce the skin. Where skin towels are placed over uneven contours requiring attachment at many places, anchoring with sutures or using stick-on drapes will eliminate the bulk of many clips. After removing towel clips at the end of a procedure, spread out the pinch marks to prevent a permanent pinched-up defect in the skin.

Stick-on Drapes

Plastic stick-on drapes may have some advantage for protecting the sterility of wounds. They are useful for draping uneven surfaces and are superior for keeping field towels from slipping, where, because of the use of local anesthetic or other reason, towel clips are undesirable. A single person can apply stick-on drapes. The technique is shown in Figure 151. After peeling back two inches of drape covering on one edge, hold the unrolled protective covering in your right

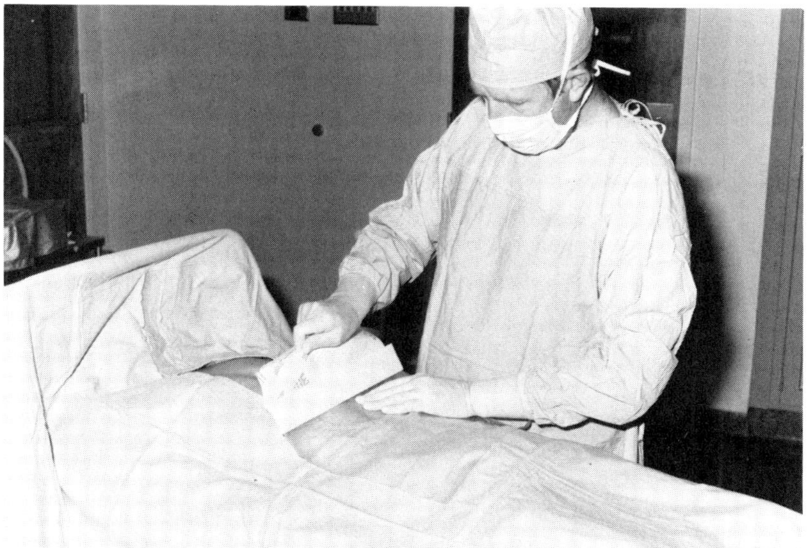

Figure 151. To apply stick-on drape, peel back an inch or two of drape covering from one edge, hold the unrolled protective covering in the right hand, while the left hand presses the exposed end to one margin of the operative field.

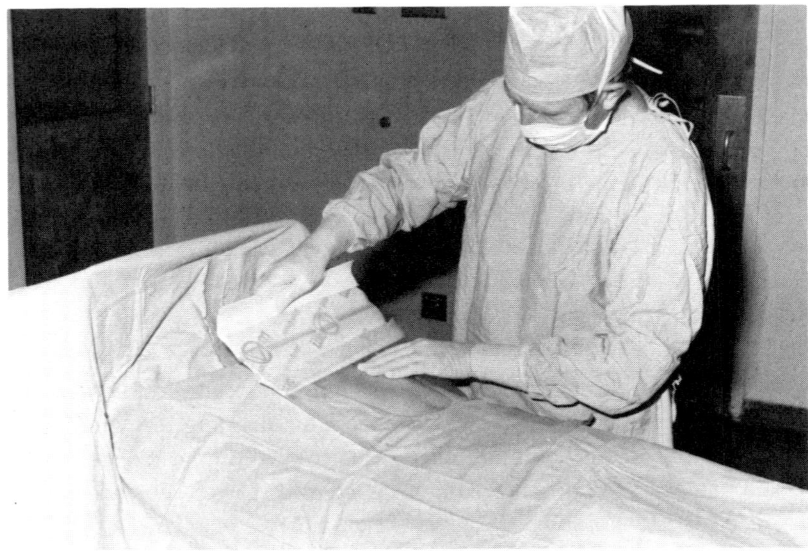

Figure 152.   With the left hand, spread, smooth, and press the stick-on drape in place, as the right hand completes the separation of the drape from its protective covering.

hand. With your left hand press the exposed end to one margin of the operative field. Now, spread, smooth, and press the drape in place with your left hand as you unroll and separate the drape from the remainder of its protective covering with your right hand (Fig. 152). The one-person technique of drape application is superior, especially when used over uneven surfaces, where the exposed portions of adhesive can be applied while protecting the remainder from inadvertent undesirable attachment. The drape is unrolled while pressing each newly exposed area of adhesive evenly into depressions and over lumps.

Chapter 10

Operating Room Personnel

Among the most important tools available to a surgeon are the hands of others. In the metamorphosis of a student into a polished surgeon, the full coordinated use of assistants and other operating room personnel remains the last step to be mastered. To maintain control of an operation, the surgeon must control the activity of people around him. He has a choice of two methods to maintain dominance: He may terrorize his helpers into submissive behavior, or he may lead by gaining their respect and confidence which will, in turn, produce the desire to cooperate in their joint effort.

The first method, that of fear, is a cheap and easy method resulting in decided advantage to the inferior surgeon, since the terrorized people become so preoccupied with their own anxieties over their inability to fulfill that surgeon's demands that the incompetence and mistakes of the surgeon go unnoticed. In fact, he may convince the operating room personnel that they are to blame for his failures. Strangely, abused operating personnel become very loyal to their surgeon, much like an abused child is loyal to his parents. Thus, terrorization of the operating room staff remains a cheap shot found very useful by incompetent surgeons. A modern surgeon should acquire the scientific knowledge, technical skill, and personality competence that make it unnecessary for him to hide his inadequacies by terrorizing the people around him.

The surgeon who is terrorizing his operating personnel is manifesting his incompetence.

The second method of operating-room leadership, that of the surgeon's inspiring his helpers with respect and confidence in him, is tough, yet very rewarding to the patient as well as to the surgeon and his associates. Competent leadership of an operating room starts with the surgeon's gaining control of his own personality. The development of useful personal traits can be practiced and perfected just as skills can be developed with any of the other tools.

The surgeon who removes a patient's bleeding duodenal ulcer while helping to create one in his anesthetist or nurse is not really a humanitarian.

One of the most useful personality traits in a surgeon is imperturbability. Many critical situations arise where the success of an operation is inversely proportional to the irascibility of a surgeon. If a surgeon keeps his "cool" instead of becoming hysterical in emergency situations, his team performs with maximum efficiency. Members of the surgical team always know when crises exist; therefore, there is no need to inform them by yelling, pleading to our Maker, or screaming obscenities. Instead, a calm request for the necessary instruments and tools, with the admonition to take enough time and do it accurately, will get utensils to you immediately. A student can hold a clamp steadier, a nurse can thread a needle faster or get a critical instrument quicker, if told "do it right" rather than a panicky "hurry, hurry, hurry."

Imperturbability can aid in the handling of critical massive bleeding where, instead of yelling for vascular clamps, gentle pressure placed at the bleeding site will allow the necessary time to calmly assess the situation, increase the exposure, get the proper tools and equipment ready, and thereby turn what might be a frantic emergency situation into a controlled event. Self-control is the starting point for gaining control of others.

Success in critical surgery is inversely proportional to the irascibility of the surgeon.

THE USE OF ASSISTANTS

Have a Detailed Plan

In order to use an assistant to the fullest advantage, a surgeon needs a detailed step-by-step plan of the operation. The plan must include the steps that the surgeon performs and also what he wants his assistants to do. There is, of course, no way of directing the activity of an assistant if you do not know what you want him to do.

If a surgeon has no plan or method of obtaining exposure, his operation quickly becomes altered by the whims of his assistants. If the assistant is a dominant personality with methods of his own, the surgeon can soon be led through the procedure by steps that are not preconceived by him, and his activity may not be preconceived by the assistant. The end result is different from that envisioned by either. A hodgepodge of inefficiency results, and the operation just happens instead of having been performed with direction and control.

Don't let the operation just happen.

To use assistants, your plan must include every detail of every step of the operation: who ties each knot, where you want sponges and retractors placed, which assistant holds each structure or tool, and which hand is used in each instance. The less that is left to the judgment of others, the more you can predict and control the surgical result, and the more efficient your operation will become.

A well-planned operation makes an assistant look good. A poorly planned operation needs a skilled assistant with his own plan to make a surgeon look good.

Brief Your Assistants Preoperatively

Before entering the operating room, brief your assistants on the steps of your procedure and the role you expect each to play. There will not be enough time to describe your technique during the course of the operation, because maneuvers that require a mere few seconds to perform frequently take a minute or two to describe and explain. Conversation during the 10-minute scrub may be sufficient briefing time for relatively uncomplicated procedures. A well-briefed assistant, knowing what you intend to do next, will not need to be psychic to provide good help, and may better suppress his desire to improvise during your operation.

Ironically, the more experienced an assistant, the more important the briefing. In the operating room an inexperienced medical student will do exactly as he is directed by the surgeon and will take no liberties. However, an unbriefed colleague may try to impose his methods on your operation. This paradox is most acute when a senior surgical resident plans a procedure in every detail and is then assisted by a senior attending surgeon without preoperative discussion between the two. The attending surgeon constantly imposes variations different from the resident's plan, while the resident's planned steps continue to distort the attending surgeon's efforts. The result is a shambles that neither of them planned, and is accompanied by a loss of confidence in each other.

If your assistant is an experienced surgeon, to dominate him you must brief him well. If you cannot dominate him, select another assistant the next time you need one, as surgery should be performed by compatible people.

Pick an assistant that you can control.

Don't Oscillate the Assistant's Functions

It is inefficient for an assistant to interrupt his performance of an important static function to do some trivial chore for the surgeon or another assistant. For example, if an assistant is maintaining good exposure, and lets the exposure collapse so he can tie or cut a knot that could have been handled by you or someone else, this wastes the time necessary to regain the exposure. With a well-planned operation avoid assistants' changing jobs without your direction.

Have the Patience To Let
an Assistant Finish His Step

Whenever the surgeon is idle, waiting for an assistant to finish his step in progress, there is an almost uncontrollable urge to take the step away from him. Patience to wait for an assistant is a rare commodity, rewarded by improved efficiency and time saving. If an assistant is untangling two ends of a ligature to be tied by the surgeon, who at that moment has nothing else to do but wait, we frequently see impatience. The surgeon will grab the almost untangled ends away from the assistant, retangling them and negating the order and progress the assistant has already made. If an assistant is preparing suture ends for you, waiting for him will save time in the end. You don't have to be active all the time the operation is in motion. It is essential for a surgeon to be idle some of the time if he is taking full advantage of his assistants. Let the assistant perform his maneuver.

Impatient surgeons, instead of remaining idle, frequently waste time by taking away a step which an assistant already has in progress.

Don't Assist Yourself

In the development of our surgical experience we start as assistants, then eventually become surgeons. During the transition, a neophyte surgeon frequently resists giving up his well-learned job of being an assistant as he adds the new duties of a surgeon. For example, when a new surgeon who has been tying and cutting sutures gets to do the sewing he frequently insists on also continuing the cutting and tying, which should now be relegated to his assistant. His failure to assign these duties requires that he interrupt his sewing, change instruments from needle holder and forceps to ties, to scissors, and back again, wasting time that could have been saved by an assistant. Much time is wasted by surgeons who insist on assisting themselves.

Don't assist yourself.

Have Only One Person Doing Each Job

Duplication of activity is obviously a waste; but duplicated effort is not the only waste. The time that could have been expended on another important task is also wasted. For example, if a surgeon cauterizing small bleeders has a sponge in one hand and his assistant, too, has a sponge, the double sponging is not the only waste. One hand could have been freed to maintain better exposure. A surgeon's hand retracting one side of the wound and the assistant's hand retracting the other side, the assistant sponging and the surgeon cauterizing, is better use of the four hands than two sponges with less exposure.

Develop a Better Vocabulary for Communication

A minor well-conceived expansion of vocabulary will allow a surgeon to communicate with his helpers with less misunderstanding. It is an ambiguous instruction, for example, to tell an assistant placing a stitch to "take a bigger bite." Such a request could mean: make more progress between stitches; make a wider cuff; or take a thicker cuff of tissue. Planning a vocabulary that will allow you to communicate by nonambiguous, specific instructions will greatly facilitate coordination between surgeons and assistants.

"Four-letter words" are too nonspecific to be effective in communicating anything other than displeasure.

The Use of Instrument Nurses, Circulating Nurses, or Technicians

Many of the principles applicable to using assistants also apply in dealing with instrument nurses and circulating personnel. The preoperative briefing should involve not only having a written card for tools and equipment for standard procedures, but some verbal communication with reference to special instruments if variations from the standard case are to occur.

There is great advantage for the surgeon to check the equipment table before scrubbing, to keep from being surprised after an incision is made. It is embarrassing to find no cardiac pacemaker in the hospital after a pacemaker pouch is already constructed; or to have a bronchoscopic exposure of an endobronchial tumor before discovering that the biopsy forceps have been broken and the available one is shorter than the bronchoscope. The assembly of tools and materials may be delegated to operating room personnel, but verification of the presence of necessary equipment before starting an operation remains the responsibility of the surgeon.

Briefing the instrument nurse preoperatively with a general description of the procedure and allowing her to see the field during the operation, will result in better assistance during subsequent similar operations. Also, isolation from the field doesn't engender a good feeling of involvement.

The development of a vocabulary to communicate with the instrument nurse requires that the surgeon know the names of instruments, caliber and lengths of suture materials, and specific designations of needles. Specific requests for instruments result in more rapid tool delivery. Pet names for a few favorite often-used tools may avoid confusion when one is working with the same crew day after day. A little thought will allow development of a very specific vocabulary for communicating how you want tools passed, such as "backhand the needle, hook the needle, or place the needle at midshaft" will make surgery go much more smoothly.

Preoperative instructions to the instrument nurse on how you want instruments to be passed will allow you to be more efficient and will increase the enjoyment of your work. If you do not like to have instruments popped into your hand as seen on television, preoperative instructions will prevent irritation and bad feelings caused by complaining during the procedure. Good interpersonal relationships result from solving problems before they happen; prevention is less of an affront than a complaint.

Much time is wasted in the operating room by surgeons who wait until they need an instrument to request it. If you call for tools one step ahead, you will not have to wait for them. Constantly notify the operating personnel of the tools used in the next step so they can anticipate your need.

Think, plan, and request ahead.

Pass the unused instruments back to the instrument nurse. Hoarded instruments not only clutter the field, but make them unavailable for redelivery by the nurse upon your request.

Make specific requests of specific persons to avoid misunderstanding and nonperformance. Nonspecific requests may leave everyone thinking the other person is carrying out the order.

In an emergency room situation a loud request to "get ten units of blood typed and cross-matched for this patient" may be followed by three people leaving the room. All remaining assume that someone has gone for blood. The truth may be that two have gone to lunch and one has completed his shift and is going home. No one has gone for blood. Pointing to someone, or calling his name, while saying, "You are responsible for getting ten units of blood," "You do the cut down," "You get me a chest spreader," "You get me a laparotomy set," lessens the confusion, avoids misunderstanding, and creates order out of what would otherwise be chaos. Give specific orders to specific persons.

A person leaving the operating room, whom you think is responding to your nonspecifically aimed "go for" request, may, in reality, be going out to lunch.

Communication is a two-way street. Be sure to acknowledge that you have heard such reports as, "The sponge count is correct." Otherwise, you may give the impression that you are not interested, and the important reports will cease.

Utilizing the Anesthesiologist

The anesthesiologist is a partner in surgical procedures. Discussion of each case is essential for coordination that will ensure optimal patient care. Including the anesthesiologist in a preoperative discussion will allow incorporation of his knowledge into a better plan. A feeling of cooperation rather than competition is essential for best results.

There is no place for the isolation characterized by the answer to one surgeon who asked his anesthetist, "How is the patient doing?," and was told, "You take care of your side of the ether screen and I will take care of mine." Letting the anesthesiologist know in advance when there will be blood loss allows him to handle replacement sooner and without urgency. A reliable estimate of an operation's duration will let him plan the anesthetic to the patient's best advantage. Plans for I.V. lines to be used postoperatively and anticipated postoperative respiratory support should be discussed in advance.

INTERRELATIONSHIP OF TEAM MEMBERS

Besides a surgeon's controlling his own interpersonal relations with members of the operating team, he should maintain some control over interpersonal relations of members among themselves. Above all else, the surgeon should not let interpersonal problems among members of the operating room staff turn the operating room into a battlefield. The surgeon should insist that they do their fighting before or after, but not during, the operative procedure. If a surgeon is skillful in dealing with his associates and helpers, the operating room can be an enjoyable place rather than the hospital battlefield.

The operating room should not be a battlefield of domineering surgeons and their alienated team members.

COMMON COURTESY

For conservation of time we omit "Please" and "Thank you" during an operation, but good manners require acknowledgment at the end of the procedure of the expert help one has received. Building effective relationships with one's team members is aided by verbal follow-up reports of interesting cases. The awareness of accomplishment will increase the O.R. team's interest and performance.

Chapter 11

*Perspectives on Sutures**

Standards for sutures were first included in the United States Pharmacopeia (USP), an official compendium with its standards mandatory under federal law for products so labeled, in 1937. USP XX monographs describe Absorbable Surgical Sutures and Nonabsorbable Surgical Sutures. Standards and tests are given for suture size, diameter limits, and tensile strength. In addition, USP suture standards cover suture packaging, labeling, needle attachment, dyes, and sterility. Prior to 1976, some sutures were categorized as "drugs" for regulatory purposes under the Food, Drug, and Cosmetic Act of 1962. With burgeoning use of complex diagnostic and therapeutic equipment, the Medical Device Amendments of 1976 were enacted to provide greater consumer protection. Under this legislation, sutures are classified as medical devices, and manufacturers are required to submit substantial proof of suture safety and efficacy to the Federal Food and Drug Administration.

*© DAVIS + GECK, 1980.

USP XX AND SUTURE STANDARDS

USP XX standards for sutures must be met by manufacturers if their product labels indicate that they conform to the compendial standards. If questions arise concerning suture properties, it is the USP standards against which the product will be judged.

USP XX carries this description of absorbable surgical suture:

Flexible strand varying in treatment, color, size, packaging, and resistance to absorption, according to the intended purpose. The collagen suture is either Type A Suture or Type C Suture. Both types consist of processed strands of collagen, but Type C Suture is processed by physical or chemical means so as to provide greater resistance to absorption in living mammalian tissue.

Absorbable Surgical Suture is a sterile strand prepared from collagen derived from healthy mammals, or from a synthetic polymer. Its length is not less than 95.0 percent of that stated on the label. Its diameter and tensile strength correspond to the size designation indicated on the label, within the limits prescribed herein. It is capable of being absorbed by living mammalian tissue, but may be treated to modify its resistance to absorption. It may be modified with respect to body or texture. It may be impregnated or coated with a suitable antimicrobial agent. It may be colored by a color additive approved by the Federal Food and Drug Administration.

The diameter of each suture strand must fall within the minimum and maximum limits for its gauge. These limits differ for collagen and synthetic absorbables (Tables 1 and 2). Metric size designations are now included along with USP size (gauge) to facilitate voluntary international uniformity in suture standards. USP also sets standards and tests for packaging, labeling, needle attachment, dyes, and sterility. USP XX provides this description of nonabsorbable surgical suture:

Flexible, monofilament or multifilament, continuous strand, placed in an envelope, tube, or other suitable container or wound on a reel or spool. If it is a multifilament strand, the individual filament may be combined by spinning, twisting, braiding or any combination thereof.

Nonabsorbable Surgical Suture is classed and typed as follows: Class I Suture is composed of silk or synthetic fibers of monofilament, twisted, or braided construction. Class II Suture is composed of cotton or linen fibers or coated natural or synthetic

TABLE 1: USP Specifications for Collagen Suture

USP Size	Metric Size (Gauge No.)	Limits on Diameter (mm)		Limits on Knot-pull Tensile Strength (kg)
		Min.	Max.	
	0.01	0.001	0.009	
	0.1	0.010	0.019	
	0.2	0.020	0.029	
9-0	0.3	0.030	0.039	0.023
	0.4	0.040	0.049	0.034
8-0	0.5	0.050	0.069	0.045
7-0	0.7	0.070	0.099	0.07
6-0	1	0.10	0.149	0.18
5-0	1.5	0.15	0.199	0.38
4-0	2	0.20	0.249	0.77
3-0	3	0.30	0.339	1.25
2-0	3.5	0.35	0.399	2.00
1-0	4	0.40	0.499	2.77
1	5	0.50	0.599	3.80
2	6	0.60	0.699	4.51
3	7	0.70	0.799	5.90
4	8	0.80	0.899	7.00

TABLE 2: USP Specifications for Synthetic Absorbable Suture

USP Size	Metric Size (Gauge No.)	Limits on Diameter (mm)		Limit on Knot-pull Tensile Strength (kg)
		Min.	Max.	
12-0	0.01	0.001	0.009	
11-0	0.1	0.010	0.019	
10-0	0.2	0.020	0.029	
9-0	0.3	0.030	0.039	0.045
8-0	0.4	0.040	0.049	0.07
7-0	0.5	0.050	0.069	0.14
6-0	0.7	0.070	0.099	0.25
5-0	1	0.10	0.149	0.68
4-0	1.5	0.15	0.199	0.95
3-0	2	0.20	0.249	1.77
2-0	3	0.30	0.339	2.68
1-0	3.5	0.35	0.399	3.90
1	4	0.40	0.499	5.08
2	5	0.50	0.599	6.35
3 and 4	6	0.60	0.699	
5	7	0.70	0.799	

fibers where the coating forms a casting of significant thickness but does not contribute appreciably to strength. Class III Suture is composed of monofilament or multifilament metal wire.

Nonabsorbable Surgical Suture is a strand of material that is suitably resistant to the action of living mammalian tissue. Its length is not less than 95.0 percent of that stated on the label. Its diameter and tensile strength correspond to the size designation indicated on the label, within the limits prescribed herein. It may be nonsterile or sterile. It may be impregnated or coated with a suitable antimicrobial agent.

Nonabsorbable Surgical Suture may be modified with respect to body or texture, or to reduce capillarity, and may be suitably bleached. It may be colored by a color additive approved by the Federal Food and Drug Administration.

See USP specifications for nonabsorbable surgical sutures in Table 3.

TABLE 3: USP Specifications for Nonabsorbable Surgical Sutures

USP Size	Metric Size (Gauge No.)	Limits on Diameter (mm) Min.	Limits on Diameter (mm) Max.	Limits on Knot-pull Tensile Strength (kg.)[*] Class I	Limits on Knot-pull Tensile Strength (kg.)[*] Class II	Limits on Knot-pull Tensile Strength (kg.)[*] Class III[†]
12-0	0.01	0.001	0.009	0.001	—	0.002
11-0	0.1	0.010	0.019	0.005	0.004	0.017
10-0	0.2	0.020	0.029	0.016	0.012	0.05
9-0	0.3	0.030	0.039	0.036	0.024	0.06
8-0	0.4	0.040	0.049	0.06	0.04	0.11
7-0	0.5	0.050	0.069	0.11	0.06	0.16
6-0	0.7	0.070	0.099	0.20	0.11	0.27
5-0	1	0.10	0.149	0.40	0.23	0.54
4-0	1.5	0.15	0.199	0.60	0.46	0.82
3-0	2	0.20	0.249	0.96	0.66	1.36
2-0	3	0.30	0.339	1.44	1.02	1.80
1-0	3.5	0.35	0.399	2.16	1.45	3.40
1	4	0.40	0.499	2.72	1.81	4.76
2	5	0.50	0.599	3.52	2.54	5.90
3 and 4	6	0.60	0.699	4.88	3.68	9.11
5	7	0.70	0.799	6.16	—	11.4
6	8	0.80	0.899	7.28	—	13.6
7	—	0.90	0.999	9.04	—	15.9
8	10	1.00	1.099	—	—	18.2
9	11	1.100	1.199	—	—	20.5
10	12	1.200	1.299	—	—	22.8

[*] The limits on knot-pull tensile strength apply to Nonabsorbable Surgical Suture that has been sterilized. For nonsterile Sutures of Class I and Class II, the limits are 25% higher.

[†] The tensile strength of sizes larger than metric size 3 or monofilament Class III (metallic) Nonabsorbable Surgical Suture is measured by straight pull.

ABSORBABLE SURGICAL SUTURE

Absorbable sutures are broken down by body tissues, either by enzymatic activity or by hydrolysis, and they eventually disappear. DAVIS + GECK manufactures two types of absorbable sutures: DEXON® "S" polyglycolic acid suture, a synthetic absorbable, and surgical gut, an absorbable suture of animal origin (Table 4).

DEXON® "S" polyglycolic acid sutures

Polyglycolic acid (PGA), a synthetic polymer of glycolic acid, is also produced during normal body metabolism as hydroxyacetic acid. PGA is

TABLE 4: DAVIS + GECK Absorbable Suture Materials

Generic Name	Trade Name	Raw Material	Construction and Handling Characteristics	Frequent Uses
Polyglycolic acid suture	DEXON ® "S"	Glycolic acid	Very smoothly braided uncoated. Tensile strength surpassed only by steel. Excellent "hand" and knot security. Elicits mild tissue response; not violent tissue reaction. Completely absorbed.	Widely used for peritoneal, fascial, subcutaneous, and subarticular closures. Also for ligatures. Particularly well-suited for ophthalmic, plastic, and neurologic surgery. Superior strength for orthopedic applications. Completely replaces plain and chromic gut.
Surgical gut suture		Plain and chromic sheep or beef intestine	Digested by enzymes produced by inflammatory process. Weaker than DEXON "S" suture in same gauge. Twisted construction.	Use where long-term support is needed. Absorption may vary depending on patient, tissue type, and other factors.

the first material developed through modern chemical technology specifically for use as surgical suture. A man-made material, DEXON® "S" contains no collagenous protein, no antigens or pyrogens. Diameter and tensile strength can be closely controlled, producing uniform strands of greater strength than equivalent gauges of surgical gut. Tissue response is very mild when compared to the more violent, inflammatory reaction provoked by surgical gut. Hence, patient discomfort during the healing period is minimal with DEXON "S." Available sterile only, DEXON "S" is offered in natural beige or a distinctive green for visibility.

DEXON "S" is absorbed by hydrolysis during wound healing. It is completely metabolized; by-products are excreted by the urinary, digestive, and respiratory systems. Clinical experience confirmed by animal studies revealed no absorption of DEXON "S" sutures 7 days after surgery, minimal absorption at 15 days, maximum absorption at 30 days, and essentially total resorption at 60 to 90 days postoperatively. Thus, DEXON "S" can be depended upon to support the wound with optimum strength during the critical early healing period, the first 7 to 10 days after surgery.

The tensile strength of DEXON "S"—both straight pull and knot pull—compares favorably with that of the strongest nonmetallic sutures. Since its "out of package" strength surpasses that of surgical gut, DEXON "S" retains more tensile strength after tying to secure tissue. The in vivo tensile strength retention of DEXON "S" differs considerably from that of chromic gut. Laboratory studies indicate that about 46 percent of the day zero tensile strength of DEXON "S" remains after 21 days of subcutaneous implantation in rats.

The braided construction of DEXON "S" gives the strand a flexible "hand" similar to surgical silk. The tight, smooth braid passes easily through the most flexible tissue and provides the surgeon with better knot tying characteristics. On removal from the package, the strand does not coil or tangle. It resists fraying and breakage and does not become slippery during use. DEXON "S" is ready for immediate use because it is dry and sterile; no premoistening or straightening is necessary. Opened, unused strands cannot be resterilized and must be discarded.

The uncoated, braided construction of DEXON "S" assures superb knot security. Hence, the suture must be precisely tied. The surgeon's "double throw," the most proven method, assures that the first throw stays where placed, allowing subsequent throws to be run down *without* having to put tension on the first throw to hold it down. This technique eliminates potential "chatter" at run down and assures exact tissue apposition.

With few exceptions, DEXON® "S" may be used in any surgical situation in which absorbable material is indicated. This suture is in broad use in the repair of most types of surgical incisions and in ligation of blood vessels. It has been successfully used in contaminated wounds because its loss of tensile strength and rate of absorption are not affected by infection as surgical gut may be. DEXON "S" is appropriate for use in general surgery, in most specialty procedures, and for most types of wound closure. Its natural beige color cannot be seen below or near the skin surface. The predictable and uniform absorption rate and minimal tissue response of DEXON "S" make it a logical choice in ophthalmic procedures, such as cataract and strabismus surgery. It is also widely used in OB–Gyn surgery, orthopedic surgery, urologic surgery, plastic and reconstructive surgery, and most other procedures in which eventual absorption of suture is desirable.

DEXON "S" should not be used in circumstances requiring extended or permanent suture support of tissues. For example, its use is contraindicated for suturing heart valves and vascular prostheses which depend on permanent suture support. The safe use of PGA in cardiovascular and neural surgery has not been established.

Surgical Gut Suture

DAVIS + GECK surgical gut is made from healthy mammalian intestinal tissue, which, after initial processing, becomes a purified protein called collagen. The collagen is stretched and slit into long ribbons, which, after inspection for color and condition, will become either plain or chromic gut. Ribbons slated for chromic gut are bathed in a chromic salt solution before they are spun into a strand to increase resistance to digestion by tissue enzymes.

Strand size is determined by the number and width of the ribbons it contains. The desired number of ribbons are spun into a strand under carefully regulated tension, then dried in a controlled environment, cut into appropriate lengths, and inspected. Electronic sorting places them in the correct diameter group, while electronic polishing and gauging insures uniform diameter along their entire length. For surgical gut needled suture, the appropriate needle is swaged to the strand. Collagen sutures undergo sterilization by a dry heat and liquid ethylene oxide process, as well as a series of bacteriologic tests to confirm sterility. DAVIS + GECK does not release a suture production lot until USP requirements have been met. Knot strength is substantially above USP specifications.

Surgical gut must be packaged in a minimal amount of conditioning fluid to maintain pliability, and is in optimum handling condition immediately upon its removal. Gut should be allowed to remain in the packet until needed; it becomes wiry when dried out. Pliability can be restored by momentary immersion in sterile tepid water or saline.

Proteolytic enzymes absorb plain gut more rapidly than chromic gut. Factors, such as the type of tissue in which gut is implanted and the condition of the patient, affect the rate of absorption. Serous and mucous membranes, for example, absorb gut faster than do muscle tissues; while in undernourished, debilitated, anemic, or elderly patients, absorption may be faster than desired. The size of surgical gut does not significantly affect its absorption. Smaller gauges maintain tensile strength and integrity as long as the larger sizes, and provoke less tissue reaction.

Surgical gut is used in areas contraindicated for nonabsorbable sutures: kidney, ureter, urinary bladder, and gallbladder. Although its use in infected areas is preferable to that of silk or cotton, a shorter-than-normal absorption time must be anticipated. It should not be used when long-term suture support of tissues is required. In the presence of infection, or debilitating disease, it is used only with full knowledge that absorption may occur more rapidly than usual.

NONABSORBABLE SURGICAL SUTURES

Nonabsorbable sutures remain embedded in body tissues unless surgically removed, becoming encapsulated in fibrous tissue during wound healing. DAVIS + GECK manufactures synthetic, natural fiber, and metallic nonabsorbables (See Table 5, pp. 192–3).

Synthetic Nonabsorbable Sutures

The preferred sutures for long-term support, synthetic nonabsorbables retain tensile strength even after prolonged implantation in tissue. Of the commonly used synthetic nonabsorbable sutures, the polyesters are considered to have the highest tensile strength.

***TI·CRON®** silicon treated braided polyester fiber sutures.* TI·CRON sutures are made from polyethylene terephthalate. Pellets of this synthetic polymeric are melted, extruded into fine filaments, then stretched and twisted into yarn which is braided to specific suture diameters; the gauge determines the number of strands braided together. The finished strands, left white or dyed blue, receive a unique silicone treatment (patented by DAVIS + GECK), which results in a smoothness and suppleness unexcelled in polyester sutures.

TI·CRON sutures are notable for low reactivity in tissue, high tensile strength even after prolonged periods in situ, and smooth passage through tissue. Knot tying is easy, since there is virtually no "chatter" on knot run down. Because of the extraordinarily smooth surface, knots must be made with sufficient throws to achieve security. The distinctive light blue color makes the sutures easy to see during surgical procedures. In heart valve implantation, blue and white sutures are often alternated to facilitate identification of suture ends.

TI·CRON sutures are widely used in cardiovascular and general surgery, in hand and orthopedic surgery, and in ophthalmic surgery, particularly in eye muscle and retinal detachment procedures. They are well suited for suturing prosthetic devices, such as heart valves, vascular grafts, and silicone joint prostheses.

***DACRON* braided polyester fiber sutures.* DACRON sutures are pure polyester fibers, untreated to alter handling characteristics or capillarity. These fibers are extruded, stretched, and twisted into yarns, which are braided together to form the strand. Though somewhat rougher than the coated polyesters, knot security is more easily achieved than with untreated strands. High tensile strength is maintained even

*Trademark of E.I. duPont de Nemours Co., Inc.

TABLE 5: DAVIS + GECK Nonabsorbable Suture Materials

Generic Name	Trade Name	Raw Material	Construction and Handling Characteristics	Frequent Uses
Surgical silk		Proteinaceous thread spun by silkworm larva	Braided and siliconized. *Dry silk* stronger than wet. Do not moisten before use. Has excellent "hand," ties in secure knots.	Should *not* be used when suture permanence for life required, or in biliary or urinary tract. Contraindicated in known infected area. Widely used in ophthalmic, GI surgery, neurosurgery, General Surgery, and skin closure.
Surgical cotton		Long staple cotton fibers	Twisted construction. Handles much like silk but not as strong. *Wet* cotton stronger than dry, *do* moisten cotton before use.	Used in general closure, repair of fascia thyroid, brain, and plastic surgery, serosal layer of gastrointestinal tract. Should *not* be used in infected area.
Silicone treated braided polyester fiber suture	TI•CRON®	Polyethylene terephthalate polyester	Braided and siliconized. High tensile strength retained indefinitely in tissues. Smooth, supple in handling.	Particularly useful in implanting heart valves and vascular prostheses, hand surgery, orthopedic and ophthalmic surgery.
Polyester fiber suture	DACRON*	Polyethylene terephthalate polyester	Braided, uncoated polyester fiber; somewhat rougher and stiffer than coated. High tensile strength; low tissue reactivity; good knot security.	Cardiovascular, general, ophthalmic, and orthopedic procedures.
Monofilament nylon suture	DERMALON®	Nylon 6.6 a polyamide derived from coal, air and water	Monofilament. Strong, relatively inert and nonirritating in tissues.	Skin closure and plastic surgery. May be buried in subcutaneous layer or used as pull-cut suture. Useful in ophthalmic, microsurgery, tendon repair, and as retention suture.

Braided nylon sutures	SURGILON®	Nylon 6.6 a polyamide	Braided and siliconized. Handles like silk but is less reactive and much stronger. Excellent knot security.	May be used in place of silk with excellent results. Useful for general closure.
Linear polyethylene monofilament suture	DERMALENE®	A group of light thermoplastic synthetic resins	Monofilament with minimal elasticity. Excellent tensile strength; soft and pliable for smooth passage through tissue.	General closure, skin suture, plastic surgery, tendon repair, and vascular anastomoses.
Monofilament polypropylene suture	SURGILENE®	A linear hydrocarbon polymer	Monofilament. Smooth passage through tissues; minimal tissue reaction. Maintains tensile strength in vivo.	General closure, vascular anastomosis, skin sutures, wherever nonabsorbables are indicated (except eye). Excellent pull-out suture.
Stainless multistrand steel suture	FLEXON®	A ferrous alloy	Twisted multistrand. Exceptional strength; flexible, noncorrosive, inert. Almost no tissue reaction. Nonmagnetic and electropassive in tissue fluids. Cut only with wire scissors.	Useful in known infected areas and when minimal tissue reaction desirable. Often used to repair disruption or eviscerated wound or as retention sutures.
		A ferrous alloy	Monofilament strand. Take care to avoid kinking during handling; avoid pricking gloves.	Frequently used in orthopedic, plastic, thoracic, and restorative procedures.
Silver wire suture		Silver wire	Monofilament. Very strong, more pliable than stainless steel. Has an antibacterial quality.	For closure of dehiscence and for piercing ears.

*Trademark of E.I. duPont deNemours & Co., Inc.

after prolonged implantation in tissue. Cardiovascular, general orthopedic, and ophthalmic surgeons are principal users of these strong, nonreactive, nonabsorbable sutures, available in blue or white.

SURGILON® *silicone treated braided nylon sutures.* These sutures are made from nylon 6.6, a polyamide material derived from coal, air, and water. The polyamide fiber is extruded, twisted into yarn, and braided into strands of various diameters, which receive the patented DAVIS + GECK silicone treatment. The suture may be black or white.

SURGILON handles much like surgical silk, but is about 40 percent stronger, passes more smoothly through tissue, and is less reactive. It is available in precut lengths and with either ATRAUMATIC® needles or D-TACH® removable needles. SURGILON has the tensile strength of a polyester, but, like silk, gradually loses some strength after extended periods in vivo. These sutures have a longer flexlife than silk with less brooming of strands.

SURGILON is used when nonabsorbables are indicated, with few exceptions. Similar to silk in handling and knot security, it may be used in place of silk with excellent results and no change in technique. If long-term suture support is vital (i.e., vascular prostheses and heart valves), SURGILON, like silk, should not be used.

DERMALON® *monofilament nylon sutures.* The raw material in DERMALON is, again, nylon 6.6. The synthetic polyamide is extruded into very tough, strong, and elastic monofilament strands, which are uniformly round and noncapillary. Finished sutures are available in clear, white, blue, or black.

DERMALON sutures have excellent tensile strength and more elasticity than silk; knot pull tensile strength is substantially above USP specifications for monofilament nylon. Because it is a very smooth monofilament strand, DERMALON passes through tissue with minimal trauma. However, knots should be placed carefully with sufficient throws to achieve knot security.

DERMALON is an excellent choice for general skin closure and for many plastic surgery procedures. It can be used as a buried suture in subcutaneous tissue or as a pull-out suture in subcuticular closure. As a retention suture, its easy removal is an asset. Available in gauges as fine as 11–0, DERMALON® is useful in ophthalmic, microvascular, and peripheral nerve repair procedures.

DERMALENE® linear polyethylene monofilament suture.

Linear polyethylene, a synthetic of light thermoplastic resins, is extruded into monofilament strands for these sutures. DERMALENE is less elastic than other synthetics and provokes minimal tissue reaction. Knot pull strength is above USP specifications. These sutures pass smoothly through tissue; they are soft, pliable, and easy to handle and tie. They have been found particularly useful in plastic surgery and tendon repair procedures. Other applications include general closure and skin closure, as well as small vessel anastomoses.

SURGILENE® monofilament polypropylene sutures.

SURGILENE is made from polypropylene, a polyolefin of polymeric linear hydrocarbons. This synthetic is extruded to form smooth monofilament strands, which are available clear or pigmented with Cyan Blue (copper phthalocyanine blue).

Polypropylene strands have several important characteristics: 1) They pass through tissue or vascular prostheses with minimal drag and trauma; 2) they retain excellent tensile strength during extended periods in vivo; 3) SURGILENE elongates less under tension than other polypropylenes and recover more of their original dimension sooner when tension is removed or subsides; and 4) neither tissue nor body fluids adhere to them.

Polypropylene is a strong, smooth suture material with great resistance to flexural fatigue. Knots can be tied securely without breaking the strand. Swaged to E–Z Pass needles, SURGILENE passes through tough tissue and prosthetic materials with ease and minimal trauma.

SURGILENE provides excellent long-term suture support, and is thus frequently used to suture vascular prostheses. When delayed or retarded healing is expected or when contamination is present, closure with this suture provides dependable wound support. SURGILENE is used for general closure, skin closure, and in many of the specialties: vascular surgery, cardiac surgery, orthopedics, and pediatric surgery.

Natural Fiber Sutures

SURGICAL SILK. These sutures are made from raw silk, the proteinaceous thread spun by silkwork larvae in China and Japan. The cream or orange silk is degummed, scoured, and bleached, then braided or twisted into specific diameter strands. Most silk sutures are dyed black to enhance visibility in tissue. DAVIS + GECK uses a special sleeve and core braiding process which locks the silk strands in place to increase density. The sleeve is tightly braided around the core at a carefully controlled rate in the precise, constant atmosphere of relative humidity that is essential for uniform high tensile strength. Braided strands are soaked and stretched to align fibers, increase tensile strength, and assure uniform diameter, and then subjected to the unique silicone treatment patented by DAVIS + GECK. Handling characteristics are improved by siliconizing, capillarity is reduced, and the treated silk sutures provoke less tissue reaction. Finished strands undergo electronic inspection for frays and then are cut into specific lengths. In the case of a needled suture, ATRAUMATIC® needles are then attached. Packaging and sterlization are last. DAVIS + GECK surgical silk is available in black braided, white braided, white twisted, and black twisted, silicone treated. White virgin silk, which is bleached but not degummed or siliconized, is available in 8–0 and 9–0, and primarily is an ophthalmic product.

Although surgical silk is not digested by body enzymes, it loses substantial tensile strength after 90 to 120 days of implantation. Excellent handling characteristics and knot security have made surgical silk the standard against which other sutures are judged. It is substantially stronger than cotton or linen, but has less tensile strength than comparable sizes of synthetic sutures. The handling characteristics of DAVIS + GECK silicone treated surgical silk approach that of the "ideal suture." Most surgeons recognize these sutures as well suited to the Halsted silk technique because of their softness, smoothness in passage through even delicate tissues, and their excellent knot security. A well-made knot will not slip or untie. The surgeon can cut knot ends short and leave less suture mass in tissues. Silk is useful in most tissues except the biliary and urinary tracts and is frequently chosen for suturing in the gastrointestinal tract, brain, eye, thyroid gland, nerves, cardiovascular system, and for skin closure. It is contraindicated when infection or contamination is present.

SURGICAL COTTON.   DAVIS + GECK cotton sutures are made by tightly twisting the unusually long silky fibers of the Sea Island variety of cotton. These sutures are available in white or suitably dyed. They are smooth, free from lint, fuzz, and the frayed areas often found in commercial short staple cotton. Compared with ordinary cotton thread, surgical cotton has exceptional tensile strength and uniform diameter. Although weaker than silk, it gains about 10 percent in tensile strength when moistened just before use. Moistening also reduces the tendency of surgical cotton to cling to gloves. Like silk, its use requires meticulous aseptic and surgical technique; it should not be used in wounds of known or suspected contamination. Cotton is frequently used in fascia repair; suturing of nerves and blood vessels; thyroid, brain, and plastic surgery; and gastrointestinal anastomosis.

Metallic Sutures

STAINLESS STEEL WIRE.   These sutures are made of a ferrous alloy. To avoid corrosion of buried sutures in human tissue fluids, an exacting combination of metallic components is used to form the monofilament strand and FLEXON® multistrand twisted stainless steel wire sutures. FLEXON is exceptionally strong, noncorrosive, inert, nonmagnetic, and electropassive in tissue fluids. It has excellent tensile strength comparable to equal gauges of the strongest synthetic sutures, and is flexible, easy to tie and handle. Stainless steel wire sutures require special handling techniques. The tendency of monofilament wire to kink during use has been greatly reduced by the ROTO-GRIP® attachment needle, which swivels on the monofilament wire strand as it is passed through tissue. The ends of wire sutures must be carefully handled to avoid pricking holes in gloves. Wire knots should be square and firm, with ends cut close or turned into tissue. Wire cutters or special wire scissors should always be used to cut wire sutures.

Stainless steel wire is useful in areas of known infection and when it is desirable to avoid excessive tissue reaction. Other frequent indications are in secondary repair of wound disruption or evisceration, and as retention sutures. Well tolerated in body tissues, steel wire is frequently chosen for orthopedic surgery of ligaments, tendons, bones, and nerves; for plastic surgery, such as repair of cleft lip and palate; in hernia repair;

urologic procedures; and closure of the chest following thoracic and cardiac surgery.

SILVER WIRE.   Silver wire is soft, pliable, and easier to handle than other metallic sutures. It has an antibacterial characteristic and offers exceptionally high tensile strength. Silver wire, available in one heavy size (7), is swaged to a large ½ circle reverse cutting needle for closure after dehiscence.

SURGICAL NEEDLES

Surgical needles vary in shape, size, type of point, and suture attachment (swaged or threaded). The basic shapes include straight, ⅜ circle, ½ circle, and ⅝ circle (Figure 1). Variations include the ¼ circle for ophthalmic surgery. The thickness of the needle depends on its wire diameter.

Needle points are either taper or cutting (Figure 2). Taper point needles are used in easily penetrated tissue, such as bowel and peritoneum. Cutting edge needles are used in tough tissue, such as skin and sclera. The most commonly used cutting edge needle is called reverse

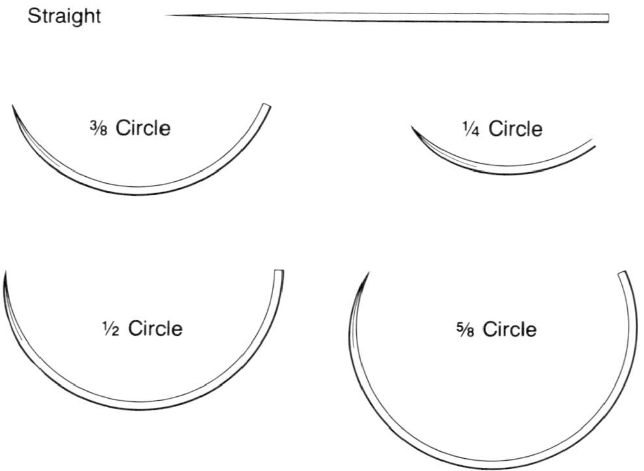

Figure 1.   Surgical needles vary in shape, size, type of point and body, and how the suture is attached (swaged or threaded).

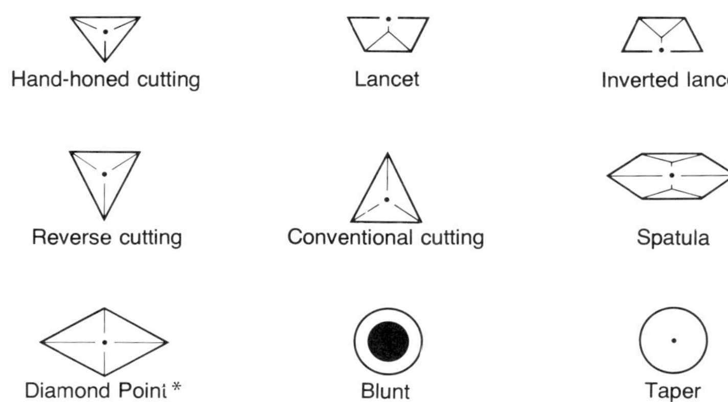

Figure 2. Needle cross sections.

cutting. Its sharp edge is on the outer curvature and appears as an upended triangle on cross section. When the inner curvature is sharpened, the needle is called conventional or regular cutting. Variations include the spatula and Lancet point for ophthalmic surgery and microsurgery. The DIAMOND POINT* is a needle with highly sharpened point and a taper body which penetrates tough tissue with ease and minimal-hole size.

To arm the needle holder correctly, the tip of the instrument is clamped at approximately one-third the distance from the swaged or eyed end of the curved needle to its point. When prepared needle sutures are placed on a flat surface, such as the Mayo tray, needle points should be *up* to avoid needle damage or puncture of the drape.

The fine needles used in microsurgical and ophthalmic procedures demand careful handling to prevent dulling or damaging their precision points and finely honed cutting edges. Fine ATRAUMATIC® needles should be considered as delicate surgical instruments and treated with appropriate care. Reusable eyed needles should be checked for burred points or rough, damaged eyes before they are threaded.

The needle holder should be passed so that the point of the needle is down—in position for the surgeon's immediate use. As the needle holder is transferred to the surgeon's hand, the scrub person controls the free suture end and hands it to the first assistant. Along with the suture, the surgeon uses tissue forceps and the first assistant requires suture

*Trademark of B.G., Sulzle, Inc.

scissors. The position of the needle on the needle holder is reversed for the left-handed surgeon, who also receives it needle point down.

ATRAUMATIC® needles

Eyeless needles, developed in 1920 and marketed under the trademark ATRAUMATIC by DAVIS + GECK, have become superior precision instruments. They provide a smooth juncture between material and needle, creating a smaller hole than threaded eyed needles. Tissue trauma and oozing are minimized (Figure 3).

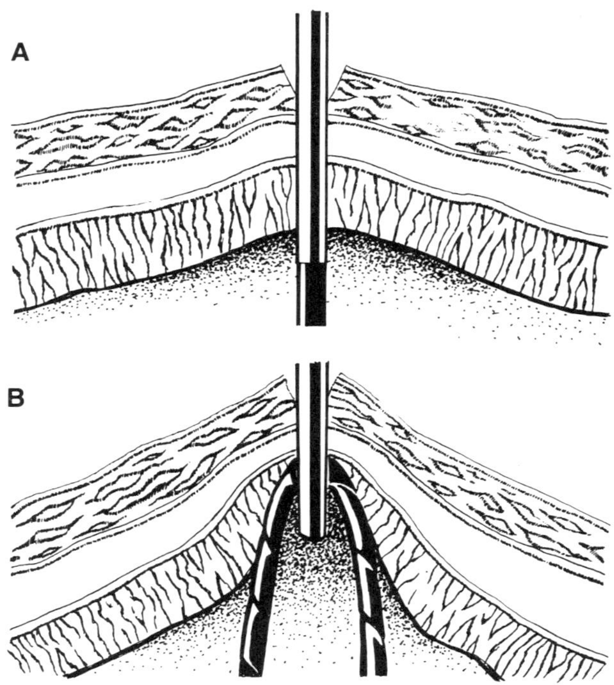

Figure 3. **A.** Drilled-end ATRAUMATIC® needles cause minimum tissue trauma by eliminating the double suture strand. **B.** Greater tissue trauma is caused by the double suture strand threaded through eyed needles.

ATRAUMATIC® needles are made of a special steel alloy, which once subjected to intensive heat and tempering under precisely controlled conditions, becomes very strong, ductile, and resistant to bending and breaking. Special equipment custom forms the steel wire into desired needle sizes and shapes. DAVIS + GECK works closely with prominent surgeons in each specialty to create new needles or modify existing ones for more effective, easier use. A full range of needle configurations, sizes, and points for every type of procedure and tissue is available.

Cutting-edge needles are honed to extra sharpness which is maintained even after repeated passes through tissue. Smooth, gradually sloping shoulders of curved ATRAUMATIC needles produce minimal holes in tissue with less chance of leakage. *Taper needles* are formed by elongating or "drawing" the wire into a slender, more tapered form than can be achieved with the grinding process used by most needle manufacturers. *Premium needles*, such as those used in ophthalmic and cosmetic surgery, require extra production techniques. Each needle body is polished and its cutting edges are meticulously hand-honed under magnification. These extremely fine, sharp needles are individually inspected and carefully protected during each phase of production and packaging. Needle ends are drilled and carefully matched to suture diameter. The surface of premium needles undergoes special treatment to increase lubricity for ease of penetration and glide through tissue.

DAVIS + GECK ATRAUMATIC needles are available in the following designs:

Conventional Cutting: Triangular with cutting edge on the inner curvature, designated by the letters SC or MC.

Reverse Cutting: Triangular with cutting edge on the outer curvature, designated by the letter C.

Hand-Honed Reverse Cutting: Triangular with cutting edge on the outer curvature specially hand-honed for fine plastic repair, designated as PR.

DIAMOND POINT:* Taper body with finely sharpened point for penetrating dense tissue but minimizing trauma, such as in car-

---

*Trademark of B.G., Sulzle, Inc.

diovascular, plastic, and ophthalmic repair, designated as DT or DG.

Spatula: Two cutting edges in the horizontal plane designed to split the tissue in thin layers, such as cornea, designated as D.

Lancet, Inverted Lancet: A variation of the Spatula Needle in which the cutting edges are on the inner (lancet) or outer (inverted lancet) curvature, designated as L for Lancet and SL for Inverted Lancet.

Straight Cutting (Keith): A straight needle with highly sharpened triangular blades used principally for skin closure and without a needle holder, designated as CS.

Straight Taper: Taper body with a straight shaft is available as ATRAUMATIC® needles or as Milliner's eyed needle. Used in interrupted closure of the skin. The ATRAUMATIC needle is designated TS-3 and 4, and the Milliner's needle TS-1 and 2.

Blunt Point: Taper body with a blunt point designed for use in soft vascular tissue such as liver, kidney, and sternal closure, designated as N or BT.

The second letter in the DAVIS + GECK needle code designated the shape: ½ circle needles have no additional letter; ⅜ circle needles are identified by the letter E (e.g., TE or CE); ¼ circle needles are identified by O (e.g., DO or CO); straight needles are identified by an S (e.g., CS or TS); ⅝ circle is identified by repeating the basic letter (e.g., TT is the designation for a ⅝ circle taper needle).

D-TACH® removeable needles

A recent modification of ATRAUMATIC needles is the D-TACH needle. The method of swaging permits the needle to be rapidly detached from the suture strand with only a light tug—a distinct advantage during rapid placement of many interrupted sutures, such as in bowel anastomosis. A variety of suture materials are available on D-TACH needles for procedures in which spring eye needles formerly were used.

ROTO-GRIP® needle attachment

ROTO-GRIP needles attached to monofilament stainless steel sutures are a unique DAVIS + GECK innovation which allows the needle to swivel 360° on the suture strand. For the surgeon, ROTO-GRIP needles reduce twisting and kinking of the wire. Because stainless steel sutures with ROTO-GRIP needle attachments are packaged in multipacks of eight sutures, fewer packages need be opened. This results in time economy for the O.R. nurse as well as less waste and greater cost savings for the hospital. DAVIS + GECK is the exclusive supplier of monofilament stainless steel with ROTO-GRIP needle attachments.

PACKAGE INSERT

82549
D3

SURGILENE®
MONOFILAMENT POLYPROLYENE SUTURE
NONABSORBABLE SURGICAL SUTURE, USP

DESCRIPTION
SURGILENE *polypropylene* Suture, (clear or pigmented) is a sterile, isotactic crystalline stereoisomer of a linear hydrocarbon polymer having essentially no unsaturation. The pigmented suture contains Copper Phthalocyanine Blue.

ACTIONS
SURGILENE causes a minimal, transient, acute inflammatory reaction. This is followed by the formation of a microscopic layer of fibrous tissue around the suture. The suture is not absorbed nor is it subject to degradation or weakening by the action of tissue enzymes.

INDICATIONS
SURGILENE may be used wherever Nonabsorbable Surgical Suture, USP is recommended. Due to its relative biological inertness, it is recommended for use where the least possible suture reaction is desired.

Because of its lack of adherence to tissue, SURGILENE is efficacious as a pull-out suture.

CONTRAINDICATIONS
There are no known contraindications.

WARNINGS
Studies to determine the safe and effective use of SURGILENE Suture in eye surgery have not been performed.

PRECAUTIONS

As with other synthetic sutures, knot security requires the standard surgical technic of flat and square ties, with additional throws if indicated by surgical circumstance and the experiences of the operator.

There is an ongoing carcinogenicity study in rats, the results of which are not yet available.

ADVERSE REACTIONS

Transitory local inflammatory reactions have been reported.

HOW SUPPLIES

Available in USP sizes, non-needled, or affixed to the various Davis + Geck AT-RAUMATIC® needles, 10/0 thru 2 for pigmented sutures; 7/0 thru 2 for clear, in one dozen and three dozen packages.

REV. 4/77

97513
DM10

DEXON® "S"
POLYGLYCOLIC ACID SUTURE
SYNTHETIC, ABSORBABLE, USP

DESCRIPTION

DEXON "S" *polyglycolic acid* Suture—Synthetic, Absorbable, USP is a homopolymer of glycolic acid, constructed of filaments finer than in an original DEXON Suture to provide optimal handling properties. The sutures are sterile, inert, noncollagenous, nonantigenic, non-pyrogenic, flexible, and braided. They are colored green to enhance visibility in tissue and are also available undyed, with a natural beige color. They are uniform in size and tensile strength, but are smaller in diameter than other Absorbable Surgical Sutures of equivalent tensile strength.

ACTIONS

When DEXON "S" Sutures are placed in tissues a minimal tissue reaction occurs, which is followed by a microscopic layer of fibrous connective tissue which grows into the suture material.

Absorption studies in animals show DEXON "S" Sutures to be equivalent to original DEXON Sutures. Studies in rabbits revealed minimal absorption at 7 to 15 days, significant absorption at 30 days, and maximum resorption after 60 to 90 days.

Tensile strength, not being a function of the absorption rate, may vary from tissue to tissue, depending in part on the rate of hydrolysis. The early tensile strength of DEXON "S" Sutures is reported to be greater than that of comparable chromic catgut. In animal studies (subcutaneous tissue in rats) it has been shown that at two weeks post-implantation approximately 55% of the original tensile strength of a DEXON "S" Suture remains. While at three weeks approximately 20% of its original strength is retained.

INDICATIONS
DEXON "S" Sutures are indicated whenever absorbable sutures and ligatures are employed.

CONTRAINDICATIONS
DEXON "S" Sutures are contraindicated where extended approximation of tissues under strain must be maintained.

WARNINGS:
The safe use of this suture in neural tissue and in cardiovascular surgery has not been established.

Under certain circumstances, notably orthopedic procedures, immobilization by external support may be employed at the discretion of the surgeon.

Do not resterilize. Discard opened, unused sutures.

PRECAUTIONS
Acceptable surgical practice should be followed with respect to drainage and closure of infected wounds.

Knot with DEXON "S" *polyglycolic acid* suture must be properly placed to be secure. Therefore, place first throw in precise position for final knot, using a double loop; tie second throw square using horizontal tension; additional throws may be used as desired.

Skin sutures which remain in place for periods of longer than seven days may cause localized topical irritation and the extended portion of suture may be snipped off after five to seven days, as indicated.

ADVERSE REACTIONS
Those reactions that have been reported include tissue reaction or inflammation, fibrous or granulation tissue wound separation and bleeding, and accumulation of fluid around subcuticular stitches.

DOSAGE AND ADMINISTRATION
Use as required.

HOW SUPPLIED
Suture sizes 8–0 through 2 dyed green and 7–0 through 2 natural beige. Supplied in cut lengths or ligating reels, non-needled or affixed to the various Davis + Geck AT-RAUMATIC® needles or D-TACH® *removable needles.* USP in one, two, and three dozen packages.

REV. 3/79

INDEX